No More Secs!

Living, Laughing, & Loving
Despite Multiple Sclerosis

A Memoir

ann pietrangelo

DEDICATION

With heartfelt gratitude to Liz, my amazing daughter. She is one of the strongest people I know and a great source of inspiration and strength; to Tommy, my younger son who threw caution to the wind in order to fulfill a dream, paving the way for me to do the same; and to David, my eldest, whose gentle prodding, insightful commentary, and unwavering support gave me the courage to tackle this project. The world is a better place with each of them in it.

My most sincere appreciation to Steve Williams, a writer and my friend, who served as deadline taskmaster and enthusiastic cheering section.

And for dearest Jim, my husband, best friend, and partner in life, with whom I laugh, cry, and live in every moment ... I love you with all my heart and soul. Your support and love are woven through every word on these pages ... and in between each line.

TABLE OF CONTENTS

CHAPTER 1
Where's My Marcus Welby Moment?

"You test results are all normal. At this point I would consider the three treatment options we spoke of. There is no hurry in making this decision, but would like to hear back from you in the next couple of weeks. If you have any questions or concerns please call me. Thanks."

When I was a kid, doctor shows were all the rage on television. I'd seen the pronouncement of diagnosis hundreds of times. The kindly old doctor touches the patient's hand and looks into his eyes as he breaks the news. He might put an arm around the patient's shoulder, or comfort the worried spouse. The camera would then zoom in on the patient's face so we can see the emotional impact up close and personal.

But it seems we're not going to get our Marcus Welby moment ... or anything that even vaguely resembles one.

The email that changes everything lands in my inbox on January 28, 2004, at 2:19 p.m. Just another email mixed with a batch of well-worn jokes and plenty of spam.

The test results are all normal. It is one of those good news/bad news situations. In this case, however, normal does not translate into a clean bill of health. It is in this instant, through this most impersonal exchange, that *normal* takes on a whole new meaning for me.

The email comes as no surprise. Diagnosis or not, life as I know it has already been altered beyond recognition. Still, the doctor doesn't actually use the words. The meaning of the email, prompting me to decide on treatment options, is clear ... but not clear enough. I want to hear the words, or at least read them. I want and need this diagnosis to somehow be declared official before I make any decisions. This is a very big deal.

The news is, for the moment, known only to the doctor and me. I fantasize briefly that if I delete the email, that if I pretend I don't know, it won't be true. If ignorance is bliss, maybe I can simply refuse to accept the information I've been given, like a child who ignores her mother's call.

Until this moment, I could still hold out hope that it was all some colossal mistake or overreaction on my part; just one of those things that happens and is soon forgotten. Sure, I've had health problems like everyone else, but nothing like this.

Even while these thoughts run through my mind, I'm aware of another stream of consciousness floating alongside. I consider these feelings as being a normal first response because, after all, nobody plans to be disabled or sick. It's just the luck of the draw and on this particular day it happens to be my turn to draw the short stick. I was never one of those "it won't happen to me" types. I'm more of a "why not me?" kind of gal. I always figure I'm as good a target as anyone else, for both bad and good life events. Now, when it's put to the test, is my chance to see if I truly subscribe to that philosophy.

My fantasy of just ignoring the news is short-lived; the realist in me wins out and I return to the task at hand. I hit the reply button and type, "Thank you. Does this mean I have a definite diagnosis of MS?" I marvel at my own matter-of-fact attitude. I am not about to let emotion rule the day and my stoic New England heritage is firmly in control.

I hear Jim's footsteps entering from the hall and dread having to tell him that our fears have been realized. I haven't had any breathing room to process this myself yet. Allowing no time to vacillate, I plunge right in.

"We got an email from the doctor," I say, and watch as he processes the news flash. His face betrays little, but he's not a hard man to understand. I swear I can see his shoulders bracing for the added weight. Our eyes lock and for a moment there is no need to speak. The long, wordless embrace does all the talking.

The afternoon passes without a reply, but I did not venture to place a call to the doctor, nor did Jim nudge me in that direction. There is no reason to rush. We've already done our homework and made a decision about a course of treatment should we receive a positive diagnosis. Another day or two will make no difference. Life can change in an instant, but our change is more like a slow-motion odyssey.

It was only a few short weeks ago that we sat in the doctor's office, waiting, while he and a colleague pored over the MRI scans we brought in with us. They walked back into the room, odd looks on their faces, and asked, "Did you even *look* at these?" They sounded almost accusatory. Of course we did. We had these scans in our possession for three months and tried in vein to make sense of the images. The neurologist who ordered the tests in the first place nonchalantly dismissed the white spots scattered throughout my brain, telling us they were nothing more than evidence of chronic migraines. But he did, in fact, look me directly in the eye when he said, "You definitely do *not* have multiple sclerosis." He made no attempt to hide his exasperation at our questioning. Repeated attacks and our own gut instincts eventually lead us to the world-renowned teaching hospital, Johns Hopkins, a two-hour commute from home.

Feeling rather sheepish at that point, we listened for the long-awaited second opinion. "These spots are clear evidence of scarring. This is MS." The scans, along with detailed patient history and neurological exam, all pointed to multiple sclerosis. "Of course, we'll have to do a series of tests to rule out other diseases, but let's go over MS treatment options while you're here." Going over treatment options sounded fairly definite.

One of the doctors grabbed a paper and pencil and proceeded to draw a graph with lines indicating the nature of relapsing/remitting MS and several types of progressive MS, and how various disease-modifying drugs may help keep me on the relapsing/remitting line of the graph. With no cure, it's all about slowing progression.

These doctors showed no trace of doubt. They'd seen this before. Today's email confirms that everything else can be ruled out and that they are confident in their diagnosis.

Even now, I don't know how one is supposed to react when told they have a chronic disease. It's definitely not the same as hearing you have a terminal disease (something that would have more clarity in years to come) but it's not exactly like hearing you have a broken bone, either.

My body is already deep in the throes of change, but my heart and mind haven't caught up to it yet.

We share dinner as usual and, later, settle in front of the television with our two kittens, a brother and sister duo named Smokey and Bandit, angling for attention while we munch popcorn. We are a little quieter than usual but it is, for all outward appearances, a typical evening in our home.

To the casual observer our reaction might appear to be a classic case of denial, but it is really more a mixture of relief and resignation, that zone you occupy after you learn something bad, but before trying to figure out how you are going to handle it. The news could have been much worse, of course, but that doesn't change the enormity of this particular turn of events.

We greet the morning with smiles and kisses and as Jim takes his place in our home office, I head across town to work and spend the morning overly engrossed in paperwork, giving no clue about my big news; all the while wondering if my email would be answered by the time I return home.

It is. The reply is brief. "Yes it does. We can talk by phone if you want to discuss it some more. Please feel free to talk to me at any time."

So that's it then. The door has closed on wishful thinking. All doubt is removed and the mystery is solved. I have multiple sclerosis. We can say it out loud now. It is no longer the mysterious stranger who we fear, but the positively identified culprit who is moving in with us, bag and baggage, to share our home and our future. We won't be strangers for long.

As for Jim and me, our already overly-complicated lives just got a little more complicated. We can look at this as one of those fork-in-the-road scenarios, but life's not really as simple as that. One decision begets another, and there's always another fork to choose. No matter which way I go, MS is coming along with me, an uninvited and unwelcome guest. Jim, on the other hand, is free to decline the invitation. He alone must wrestle with the conscious choice of whether or not to live with MS – and me. I don't envy him that process.

On this day, at least, we will move forward together, to see where this particular fork goes. To see if our bond is what we imagine it to be. To see if we can figure out how to cope with this new entity that so rudely pushed its way into our lives and into our still young relationship.

The time for talk is over, at least for today. We are alone now, each with our private thoughts as we drift off to sleep, ignoring the sounds of late night television as we snuggle together in bed, Jim's strong arms protecting me from unseen horrors.

My last waking thoughts are a jumble of emotion without form. Tomorrow morning, for the first time, I will wake up knowing that I have multiple sclerosis. Will I still be me?

CHAPTER 2
'Discombobulation' Sums It Up Rather Nicely

Jim wakes me with a gentle nudge, "Ann, time to get up."

His lips lightly brush my cheek while his left hand strokes my hair. I pretend to sleep for another 30 seconds just to let the moment last. It sure beats a screeching alarm clock. "Hmmm ... good morning."

I'm a very heavy sleeper, definitely not a morning person, but I am instantly aware of a third presence in the room. MS wastes no time in entering my train of thought.

As soon as he is certain I am fully awake, Jim exits the room with Smokey and Bandit hot on his heels in anticipation of breakfast. When I hear him making coffee, I force myself to rise, even as every instinct screams for me to pull up the covers and hide. Heading straight for the bathroom, I close the door, taking a moment to study my reflection in the mirror. Yes, I still look like me and, except for the foggy feeling from over-thinking the situation, I still feel like me. What else was I expecting?

Not long ago I was living an entirely different life, in a different home, in a different state, with a different job, and in a different body. I was just beginning to put years of upheaval and stress behind me and was looking forward to reclaiming my life. And then along comes MS to stir the pot some more.

What about Jim? Wow, talk about a bait and switch. This has got to be messing with his head as much as it is mine. Discombobulation sums it up rather nicely.

Who should we tell ... when ... and how much? There's no death sentence hanging over my head, I'm not contagious, and even any genetic link is still unclear.

This thing that, for now at least, is the main focus of our lives, actually has very little impact on anyone else. That irrational thought is back, the fear that once we put the words – "I have MS" – into the atmosphere, and people hear the news, it will become real and everything will change.

There are quite a few people in my life who have been following my saga over the past few months. They deserve an answer.

There's no doubt; I need to tell my children first. They watched with some fear as MS slowly changed me. I need to assure them that they are in no danger, and that neither am I. As teenagers, their perceptions of the world have already been challenged by their parents' prolonged and bitter divorce and by our geographical separation. How they view me and how they perceive their own futures is up for grabs once again. Being apart from them is gut-wrenching enough on its own.

My daughter, Liz, looks a lot like me, a fact that I find much more appealing than she does. When she was about four or five years old, I happened upon an old black and white photo of myself at the same age. Even I couldn't believe how similar we looked. From my facial expression to my stance, to the way I lazily draped my arm around my brother's shoulder, the resemblance was so great that when I showed it to her, she said, "Hey! That's me!"

We share many physical traits, right down to the level of our nearsightedness. MS seems to have a minor genetic link, at least as far as susceptibility, and although MS is much more common in females, her risk is still rather small. Even so, the possibility of it horrifies me. It is a fear that will continue to plague me with every health problem she encounters.

There's no need to beat around the bush. We've already talked about the possibility of multiple sclerosis, so I quickly confirm the suspicion.

Liz is, as she often reminds me, the middle child, sandwiched in between older brother David and younger brother Tommy. The trio took the news quite matter-of-factly, just as I predicted they would. Sort of like I just told them that the forecast called for snow tomorrow. They're like me in that respect and I'm not at all certain that's a good thing. They don't have any questions, but I didn't expect any today. It's just as well because I don't have any answers.

I don't relish the thought, but I have to tell their father, and do so quickly, like ripping off a bandage. Deep breath. Just the facts, ma'am, and nothing more. I hang up the phone quickly, relieved to have that task completed.

My stomach in knots, I place a call to my mother. Separated by hundreds of miles, this is a difficult piece of news to break. She's lived alone since Dad died in 1990, but my sister lives across the hall.

"Why does it have to be you? You don't deserve that." The quiver in her voice makes me want to cry.

"I'm fine, Mom, really." I can't think of anyone who does deserve it. While I did tell her about my problems and medical drama to a certain extent, I never went into the details of just how bad things really were. I didn't tell her that there were times when I could not walk, actually could not put one foot in front of the other and propel myself forward, or times when the fear in Jim's eyes mirrored my own. There didn't seem to be any point, what with the distance and all. I'm the one with the illness, but I work at comforting her, to make it sound like it's not much of a big deal. But it is a big deal to her, and after we hang up, I am left with thoughts of her all alone in her small apartment, filled with sadness for me, forever her little girl.

I can't bear to repeat this exercise again with my own siblings. It's just too much. Stealing a page from the doctor's playbook, I compose a group email.

"Just wanted to let you all know that I finally found the reason for my health problems since last summer. I have received a confirmed diagnosis of relapsing/remitting multiple sclerosis. I don't know how much or how little you all know about this, but it is not completely hereditary or contagious. I just happen to be one of the lucky ones! Wow, maybe I should play the lottery! I'm doing very well right now and deciding on treatment options. The course of MS is so different from patient to patient that it is impossible to guess. However, I'm currently feeling fairly strong and, with proper treatment, we are very optimistic about the future. I told David, Elizabeth, Thomas, and Mom already. Anyway, I just wanted to let you all know, but I want to stress that I'm fine, in good spirits, and that Jim is as supportive and helpful as can be – I'm in good hands, so no worries. Hope all is well with you."

I instantly recognize it as too cold, too formal, too matter-of-fact. It reads like a poorly written press release, and I feel stupid about sending it, but just want to be done with this business. The relative safety and comfort of the keyboard allows me to circumvent the worried facial expressions or awkward silences I imagine would be the case in a face-to-face meeting.

I haven't lived near any of my siblings since early 1982 when I moved to the Chicago area. I've lived in Virginia since 2003. Two of my brothers live in Texas, and one brother and my sister live in Rhode Island. Time and distance have done their best to keep us at arms length from each other. They should be told, but in reality, this diagnosis changes absolutely nothing for them or our relationships.

As far as I am concerned, everyone else can learn about it through the trickle-down theory. I am going to share my news at work. Ordinarily, I would not consider sharing medical information in the workplace, but very little about my life is ordinary.

I work in a funeral home, not exactly my dream job, but it's nice enough. It's family-owned-and-operated and the staff is a fairly tight-knit group. I've only been working here for three months, but it's been pretty intense. I took the job because the physical symptoms of MS, even without the official diagnosis, made it impossible for me to commute more than a few miles, or to put in a full day's work. This position came with a part-time, flexible schedule that is perfect for the time being. It is a four-mile drive from driveway to driveway. I spend most of my time doing paperwork, writing letters, and trying not to get too emotionally involved in the very serious business at hand.

It was no secret that I needed some time off to visit a specialist and that I had some kind of medical issue. I already told them I suspected MS. They've been supportive up to this point and there's no reason to think anything will change.

It didn't. No one is particularly surprised and, much to my relief, there is no pity party thrown in my honor. How MS will affect my duties remains to be seen, but my job is not crucial to the daily operation of business, so a flexible schedule should continue to suffice.

It dawns on me that these people, fairly new in my life, didn't know me when I was healthy. There is a clear before and after picture of myself that I carry in my own mind. There were people who knew me before and would notice the changes, but everyone I meet from now on will only see the after picture of me.

11

These people never laid eyes on the me who, as a child, walked at such a fast pace that nobody wanted to walk to school with me. I just couldn't seem to slow down. They didn't know the woman with a lifelong habit of staying up until the wee hours of the morning, the mother who could play piggyback and tag, or who took the stairs two at a time while carrying a basket full of laundry under one arm and fully-loaded school backpack in the other.

Bits and pieces of my life in various stages flood my senses even as visions of an unsettling future intrude.

Even as a child I remember describing strange sensations that no one understood. When I was a teen, I blamed those ridiculous platform shoes for my awkwardness. In my early 20's, I suffered extended periods of overwhelming fatigue that I didn't understand. I was told to take vitamins. How many symptoms may have been MS ... or not? Has this thing been quietly attacking me for decades? Some questions will never have answers.

I'm not sure what to make of these feelings, but I'm not sure of much right now. An emotional numbness is washing over me. Defense mechanisms are going at full throttle and I visualize iron bars popping up all around me, caging me in and protecting me from some intangible monster on the loose.

The job at the funeral home was supposed to be temporary, just until I got over whatever it was that was plaguing me. In just six months, I had three vicious MS exacerbations that resulted in near paralysis and lasted for weeks. It's too soon to know if they'll keep coming that often or if I'll have longer periods of rest in between. Maybe the treatment will help. In any case, it's going to be awhile before I can commit to a full-time job, or anything else for that matter. Just what the future holds is anybody's guess. I never gave it much thought before, but the same is true for everyone. All we know for sure, all we really ever have, is this very moment.

"I can't think about that today ... I'll go crazy if I do. I'll think about that tomorrow." My favorite Scarlett O'Hara line seems particularly fitting right now. I just want to go home and leave the world behind. I want to prepare a predictable dinner and then cozy up on the sofa with Jim and watch an equally predictable television show. I want to live out the silly little routine we've only just begun.

After months of wondering, I internalize the fact that the assault on my body is not over, will never be over. I've got to live in this body, whatever state it's in, so I'd better make my peace with it. I've got a war to fight, and I don't want any collateral damage.

What do you do when everything you know about yourself changes just as you are hitting midlife? How do you plan for life's second half with a body you've never met before? How do you cope with a relapsing/remitting disease that shows itself on some days and plays hide and seek on others, never knowing which it will be? How do you pull yourself together? I suspect I am about to discover the answers.

As my first full day after diagnosis winds to a close, I take comfort in the fact everything, arms and legs included, are fully functioning.

I have MS. *I* have MS. I have *MS*. Me. MS! Sleep comes as sweet relief.

Ann Pietrangelo

CHAPTER 3
Or He's One Hell of an Actor

Like a child at Christmas, I still get excited when the delivery truck shows up with a package with my name on it. This ordinary brown cardboard box contains a pack of dry ice inside a white Styrofoam liner. Underneath lies my first month's supply of MS medication. We eagerly open it to view the neat rows of pre-filled syringes, looking like so many soldiers poised for battle. That is exactly what they are. Come on little soldiers. Do your stuff.

I've been poked, prodded, and stuck with so many needles in the last six months that I am over any apprehension I may have once had over the nurse coming out to the house today to show me how to properly use an auto-injector.

The doorbell rings and Smokey and Bandit scatter like the wind. The woman introduces herself to us, but in my almost out-of-body state-of-mind, I can't quite grasp her name. To me, she is simply Nurse. "Well, let's see what they sent you."

We pull out the auto-injector that came with the medication and hand it over. She eyes it warily and confesses that she's never seen this particular model before, so she has to make a phone call to learn how to use it herself. We trade questioning glances as she makes her inquiries. Our confidence is underwhelming, but it can't be terribly complicated.

I take a place at the kitchen table, with Jim on one side and Nurse on the other. Bandit, affectionately known as our *big galumph* for his bull-in-a-china-shop-ways, comes back to investigate and offer a nose bump to this stranger before heading off to rejoin his sister wherever scaredy-cats hide.

Inspecting my upper arms, Nurse makes a big deal about my lack of fat. "Oh, you're so skinny … I don't know where to do it," making a face as she prolongs the word skinny, so that it sounds like an insult. She attempts to adjust the needle but is too nervous to inject my tiny arm. Good grief. Despite my polite demeanor and frozen smile, I am not amused. She asks if she can use my thigh, where I must admit, there is no shortage of fat, so I head to the bedroom to put on a robe while she chats with Jim.

It only takes me a moment to slip out of my slacks into my pink bathrobe, but when I return I find that she has already loaded the device and explained the procedure to him. I missed it? Seriously? But I'm the patient! She said it was impossible to show me now without wasting tomorrow's dose. It does not escape my notice that she directs her attention more to Jim than to me as she places the injector against the white skin of my thigh and hits the button, making a snapping sound that startles me. It stings, but it doesn't hurt much. I'd better get used to it because I'm going to have to do this every day.

Nurse tells Jim to hold a cotton ball on it if it bleeds and wraps up her obligatory little pep talk. Again, she speaks directly to Jim as though he is my parent, or keeper, or something. Am I still in the room? At 44 years old, I suddenly feel like a young child. Perhaps I'm just a little sensitive right now. No use getting upset over it. This whole situation is surreal anyway. Maybe things will look better in a few days.

Together we see Nurse to the door and head back to the kitchen. We store the medication in the refrigerator, per instructions, and put the auto-injector away in its little pouch. My thigh itches and burns and I discover a large red bump beginning to rise. I rub it gently and desperately try not to appear like I'm complaining. Just keep smiling.

We need to decide on a general time for the daily injection. I'm not a morning person, so I figure I should probably schedule the injections for evening. Jim points out that it may be easier to stick to a time frame in the morning, getting it out of the way for the day and eliminating the possibility of falling asleep before injecting. I grumble a bit at the thought of adding anything at all to my sleepy morning routine, but I do tend to nod off in the evening, so morning it is.

Jim's eldest daughter was only nine years old when diagnosed with type 1 diabetes. At that tender age, she had to learn to inject herself daily, and if she could do it, I certainly can't complain. Thankfully, she uses an insulin pump these days.

It's not my first experience with self-injections, either. Years ago a doctor gave me an auto-injector for a powerful migraine medication, but I was petrified to use it the first time. I recruited my son, David, to help me. He was just a kid, but so eager to help.

I remember how the physical agony of migraine, combined with the distress of acting weak in front of my child, set me off on a crying jag. He was braver than me and managed to get the job done anyway. It seems rather silly now.

My insurance will cover all but $50.00 of the monthly $3,000.00 this medication costs. I will receive it in 30-day increments by mail order pharmacy.

I've heard some frightening things about shopping for health insurance on the individual market with a pre-existing condition. I've lost my group coverage and am about to switch over to COBRA. It's not going to be pretty, but for sanity's sake, we must tackle one problem at a time.

We're supposed to rotate the injection site – upper arms, abdomen, lower back, and thighs. We're aiming for fat and can adjust the needle accordingly. It doesn't look too complicated. We were provided with a pamphlet and a video to familiarize ourselves with the proper technique. After dinner, I make quick work of the pamphlet and load the video.

The pretty young woman on the screen wears a smile that makes me question her sanity, and she so enjoys the process of injecting herself that I decide she is a Stepford wife for multiple sclerosis. They've got to be kidding with this.

I'm pretty sure I won't match her level of enthusiasm, and if I go around smiling like that, someone is definitely going to have me locked up.

The doctor said we should begin treatment as quickly as possible. This substance I'm injecting into myself is meant to lower the relapse rate and stave off permanent disability.

The cause of MS is unknown, although a genetic predisposition with an environmental trigger causing an abnormal immune system response is a popular theory among researchers. Sadly, there are still many more questions than answers.

There are two basic types of MS, with various subcategories. People with progressive forms of MS experience a worsening of neurologic function over time with no clear relapses. Relapsing/remitting MS, the kind that I have, manifests itself with clear-cut relapses and remissions. Remissions are blessed relief and it is my sincere desire to keep having them.

I've gathered from my voluminous reading that some people with MS go years between relapses, and many have only minor symptoms.

I seem to have started off in full-blown crisis mode – right into can't walk, can't move my arms, can't stand up straight. But I feel fine right now, almost as if nothing ever happened. Maybe this medication will slow things down. If it doesn't, well, then things might get ugly. The doctor made it clear that prognosis at this point is impossible.

Modern medicine is a wonderful thing, but it's still an inexact science. I've had my own health scares that turned out to be nothing, and agonized through several others with my children. Those experiences have taught me not to get all bent out of shape about what might be, but to deal with what is. My future is no more or less secure than anyone else's, whether they care to admit it or not.

We can handle this. We've survived the tests, some of which I am convinced are medieval torture devices in disguise. There was something called the evoked potential test, where they send electrical impulses through your limbs; the EMG, in which the doctor inserts a long needle directly into your muscles and moves it around in order to find nerve or muscle abnormalities; lots of blood work; and repeated eye exams.

And let's not forget the dreaded spinal tap, after which I needed an additional medical procedure – a blood patch – to get things back to normal. No, not the best of times.

We managed to receive a diagnosis and we've chosen a course of treatment. I've read all the literature. In fact, the pile of MS-related reading material is beginning to bug me. I've had MS up to my eyeballs and I wonder if it will ever fade into the background so that we can think about other things.

Jim is taking ownership of the situation along with me. It's apparent that he doesn't view this as my problem, but as our problem. If he harbors any resentment at all, I can't detect it. That bodes well for our future together, and I silently reaffirm my love and respect for him.

It's not that he doesn't have other things on his mind. Jim has been involved in the coin-op amusement industry for more than 20 years – coin-op, as in the jukeboxes, video games, and pool tables you might play at your local pizza parlor or arcade. As president of Interactive Digital Systems (IDS,) he is working with others to put the final touches on a system they designed that will enable them to beam, via satellite, digital files to a nationwide network of video jukeboxes. The goal is to create a highly targeted advertising network. If that isn't enough to keep him busy, he is on the board of directors of the Amusement and Music Operators Association (AMOA,) an international trade group representing much of the amusement game industry. He has been elected its next president and is preparing to take over that position at their annual fall meeting in Las Vegas. Despite working from home, Jim is a busy man.

Raised in New Jersey, Jim moved to Louisiana when he accepted a position as General Manager for a highly respected coin-op game distribution company. Six years later, the gentleman who owned the company passed away and Jim, rather than staying on with the new owner, accepted the position at IDS, moving once again, this time to Virginia. Jim has three grown daughters, each of whom have settled elsewhere with careers and families. So, like me, geography separates him from his family. Like so many parents in today's society, we've had to learn to live and work with that regret.

Jim has been wonderfully supportive, but we can't linger in this void much longer. The time has come for us to move on. The initial attacks, the stressful road to diagnosis, and the basic decisions about treatment are behind us now, and it's time to go about the business of living. Time to work and do the chores and go back to whatever it was we were doing before all the craziness began.

I'm just not sure how to get from here to there. We know that another MS attack is likely to happen. But when and how severe are questions yet to be answered. It's enough to make us appreciate the here and now.

There are no signs of hesitation on Jim's part. He's either one hell of an actor or his love for me is stronger than his aversion to MS. I'd like to believe the latter. The next few months should tell the tale and, believe me, I take absolutely nothing for granted.

Ann Pietrangelo

CHAPTER 4
The Big Drip

It didn't take long for us to fall in to a new routine. Every morning Jim takes my injection from the box in the refrigerator and leaves it on the counter to warm to room temperature.

Jim makes it a playful, even sexy part of our morning. "Come here, baby … I've got something for you …" He holds out his arms and flashes the smile that I find impossible to resist. I saunter over and he pulls me close. Beginning at my collarbone, he runs his hand slowly down to my waist and gently unwraps my robe. His gentle touch on my bare skin is so light I barely feel it, yet I am electrically charged. There is an undeniable physical chemistry at play between us.

He decides on the injection site and presses the auto-injector against my skin. Snap! He finishes up with a hug and a kiss. Mornings are looking a lot better these days. I am convinced that we are weirdly, but perfectly, compatible.

Often I don't feel the shot at all, because some parts of me are rather numb. Sometimes it's a bad sting followed by bumps and redness. Every now and then we accidentally hit a vein, which can be fairly messy. I find it goes much better if I brace myself against the kitchen counter so that I don't sway.

I'm starting to notice many minor adjustments on his part. He's a creature of habit and has incorporated my MS into his routine. "How're you doing out there babe?" he'll ask if I've been quiet too long. The laundry basket I leave at the top of the stairs magically ends up downstairs and vice versa, and he practically races me to the sink to do the dinner dishes before I have a chance. He pushes the grocery cart and carries most of the bags.

Without benefit of the spoken word, a certain rhythm, both mental and physical, has come to our relationship.

A few days ago the first inklings of impending trouble appeared. It's hard to describe the sensation because it is fluid, changing from moment to moment, from pins and needles to stabbing pain to complete numbness, and just plain strange.

I didn't want to mention it to Jim until I was sure, but it feels like the real deal now, with all four limbs weakening by the day, my gait widening considerably and my arms ungracefully flailing about in an effort to maintain balance. It is an emotional slide, this slow loss of control over my own body. As I awaken each morning, I take inventory of limbs, hoping to get mind and body in sync. They don't all necessarily work properly, but all limbs are present and accounted for. Let's roll!

The doctor made it clear that we should call when I felt a relapse coming on, so now I'm scheduled for something called a Solu-Medrol drip. It's some kind of steroid and I need to go to the hospital every day for four days in a row to get the intravenous drip, which we're told will take an hour or two each time.

Jim can't bear the thought of sending me off on this little adventure alone, so we set off for the hospital together, unsure of what to expect.

After a flurry of paperwork and minor confusions, Jim is left behind as I am whisked away without him.

There is no need for a hospital gown or anything for an IV drip. I am ushered into a large room lined with reclining chairs, a nurses' station, and a television up in the corner. Every chair has an IV pole next to it. Only a few of the chairs are occupied and I take a seat facing the television.

The nurse appears out of nowhere, "Hi. I'm Marilyn and I'll be taking care of you today. I work with multiple sclerosis patients all the time … you and I are going to be seeing a lot of each other from now on."

We are? That's news to me. No offense intended, lady, but I don't think I like the sound of that. I give her a half-hearted smile and silently wish for her to just get down to the task at hand. Let's not drag this thing out. All I can think about is that Jim should have stayed home so I wouldn't have to feel bad about him cooling his heels out there.

Mercifully, she hits my vein on the second try. My tiny veins usually give nurses fits and I generally end up bruised. She hoists the bag up on the pole and hands me a remote for the TV volume control. I answer "no thank you" to the stale magazines and "yes, please" to the offer of a blanket. It's cold in here and I'm already shivering.

My attention quickly turns to some morning talk show and a completely pointless story about some young, obnoxious celebrity or other who is heading off to rehab. It's weird to think that, rather than sitting at my desk at work, I'm relaxing in a Lazy Boy and watching daytime television. It is almost as if I've stepped into a scene from someone else's life.

I'm definitely going to recommend to Jim that he stay home tomorrow. I can handle this on my own. I start to come out of my own head and turn my attention to the other patients. Other than the television and the hustle and bustle from the corridor, the room is quiet, lacking even polite chatter.

There's an elderly man in the opposite corner. He appears rather serene, with a half-smile on his face and his eyes closed. What's his story? I'm not here on a life and death mission, but perhaps he is. Maybe it's chemo drugs in his IV, racing through his system; maybe it's not his first round; maybe he's working on positive imagery; maybe he is dying. Oh, God.

There is a middle-aged woman down the row to my left. She, too, has her eyes closed and is not looking for companionship. Does she have MS? Cancer? Is she worried about dying and leaving her children behind?

I know very little about the diseases that would cause a person to end up in this room today. What manner of horrors are these people battling and why am I intruding in their space? I feel like a fraud. It is not out of the realm of possibility that they feel the same way. Nobody wants to belong to this little club, but I'm quite certain that I am the healthiest person here. I wonder if they can see that. I wonder if they are thinking about me, too, or if they are consumed with the fight. Should I be doing some sort of mental imagery here? What am I supposed to feel?

Unbeknownst to me at this time, I will ultimately learn the answers to these questions. I will one day sit in seats like this again, hooked up to an IV, then a chemo port. I will know the quiet thoughts of a human being fighting for life and facing difficult, but life-affirming truths. The next few years will give me the fortitude and confidence to face what is yet to come.

I close my eyes and turn my thoughts to my kids. They do not need another crisis in their lives and I've got to keep things under control for their sake. And then to Jim. Good grief. He's been a trooper, but at some point, he's going to realize that I come with too much drama. This is not exactly the kind of emotion I was hoping to bring into his life.

My love for him is the kind of love I wish I understood earlier in life. There are no rose-colored glasses involved; it's eyes wide open all the way. We've accepted each other for the very real human beings we are, flaws and all. But this MS thing ... it's not a flaw ... it's more like a third wheel that we're going to have to carry around with us. I don't think he bargained on that. Fortunately for me, it's not something over which I have any control. I love him and want to share a life with him. I believe we are up to the challenge of MS. He's going to have to come to that conclusion of his own free will. It is possible that he already has. It is possible that it's not even a question in his mind. It is possible that he wants out, but doesn't know how to make his exit. I could take anything but a pity-based relationship.

One of the things I love about him is his determination to at least attempt to see an issue from every angle, to weigh the best that can happen and the worst that can happen and decide what he can live with. I silently wish him good luck with that.

A couple of hours later I rejoin Jim and he takes me home, because I've already missed most of the workday. By day three of this routine, I am a different person. I talk nonstop. Jim looks at me as I speak but I have the feeling he is only humoring me, because he can't possibly be interested in the mindless drivel pouring out of my mouth. Maybe it's like watching an accident happen, or maybe he only hears "waa waa waa waa," a la Charlie Brown cartoons. Even I can't stand the chatter, but I'm pumped and powerless to stop. I say I won't talk anymore ... and then I do. I talk about talking too much. I talk about not talking. I talk and talk and talk.

The funny part is that Jim has, at times, said that I don't talk enough. Be careful what you wish for, sweetheart. I pronounce this medicine a miracle drug as I embrace my newfound mania. I can do anything – up and down the stairs with the laundry basket and acing chores like nobody's business, I no longer have MS! I can take home the bacon and fry it up in the pan. Just hand over the magic bracelets because I am Wonder Woman! It's an amazing improvement, if not a cure, and I would greatly appreciate it if they would deliver this stuff to me in bulk.

Sleep has always come easily to me and that has, in fact, been quite a problem. But now I can't sleep. At night I stare upward, eyes wide open, brain going at full throttle. Even when I manage to close my eyes, they pop open against my will as if operated by tiny springs. I truly don't care, though, because I'm not tired and sleep is a colossal waste of time, isn't it? I've wasted too much of that already. There's so much more to be done. I think I've discovered how to get more hours out of my day. I just wish I knew what to do with them.

Jim is a light sleeper and it's impossible to get out of bed without waking him. "What's wrong?"

"Nothing. Sorry I bothered you. I can't sleep. I'm going to go watch TV or something."

Click. "Hi. BILLY MAYS, HERE!" He's shouting about a hands-free something or other so I can talk and drive at the same time. Scintillating. Click. *Leave It To Beaver.* You know, that Eddie Haskell isn't such a bad kid after all. Nothing much ever really happens on this show. This was the original show about nothing. Click. *Bewitched.* Elizabeth Montgomery was a beautiful woman and I just adored her and her witchcraft when I was a kid. I always felt bad for the second Darrin. I don't think people really gave him a chance. Click. Aw, cute little Laura Ingalls gets to me every time, but I don't want to learn any painful life lessons tonight. Click. Click. Click. Even if I land on a show I enjoy, I keep on clicking, searching for something that will hold my attention for more than a few minutes. I am one with the remote control. It is another little miracle invention!

When I was growing up, we had an old clunker of a black and white television set that had a broken channel knob. We had to change the channel with a pair of pliers, so we generally watched whatever show happened to be on. Things sure have changed. Now I am lord and master of all television. But that doesn't mean I can't read a book, too.

I leave the TV on and thumb through a John Grisham novel that I've already read. How does he manage to keep churning them out? I always know where he's going, but enjoy the ride so much that I can't resist.

Smokey and Bandit repeatedly attempt to settle in and cuddle with me, but I'm too fidgety for their tastes. 2:00 a.m., 3:00 a.m., 4:00 a.m. The hands on the clock are moving with lightening speed, just like my brain. It'll be morning soon, and time to go to work. I think I'm finally drifting off.

"How're you doin', babe? Are you going to work today?" There's a hand gently running through my hair. It's 7:30 and Jim rouses me from the deep sleep it took so long to achieve. Work? Sure, no problem. I revel in my energy and strength.

"I have MS, but it doesn't have me!" It's a saying popular among people with MS and I embrace the concept. I can beat this thing. It's not going to get me down. Ann, the Conqueror!

A few days after my last drip I discover the downside to this little miracle drug. The relapse arrives anyway and I'm crashing big time. It is a complete reversal of my previous mania. The fatigue is overwhelming and no matter how much I sleep, it's not enough. Oh, I definitely have MS, and it appears to have me. I seriously detest that saying right now. I had planned on going to work this morning, but I can't even finish my shower without stopping for a break. My arms are so weak that I can't manage to hold the blow dryer up to complete the job. My arms are outrageously heavy and fighting my commands. Alone in the bathroom, I release the pent-up sobs and let the tears flow. That I cannot complete this simple everyday task is a powerful reminder of the seriousness of multiple sclerosis, and I'm feeling fairly pathetic.

That whole steroid thing seems like more trouble than it's worth. What's the point of it? I remember the doctor saying something about long-term benefits, but right now it's hard to care about long-term anything. I feel like I've lived a lifetime just this week.

Even though I've been through these exacerbations before, the rapid repeat performance is startling. I'm on meds now, and just had a huge blast of steroids, but this relapse is having its way with me, dominating every inch of my being. MS is a formidable foe.

This time we know what is happening, but that knowledge only helps a little. The thought that this is how it's going to be from now on is something I cannot allow myself to ponder for long; the uncontrollable fatigue won't allow it anyway. I wrap myself in my robe, call in sick, and fall back into bed, wet hair and all.

I wake up again at 10:30 as Smokey playfully tugs at my hair. Jim has already eaten breakfast and is engaged in a conference call across the hall. He's got his phone on speaker so he can continue to work while he listens. He hears me groan like an old woman as I prop myself up, hits the mute button, and calls, "How're you doin' babe?"

"I'm okay, sweetheart." I'm 5' 6-1/2" tall and weigh 129 pounds, but I feel morbidly obese. My legs won't follow orders to move forward and I feel as though I'm trying to push through a wall of mud. I have somehow stepped into someone else's body, and I'm not particularly happy with the fit. It is all so unfamiliar. I want my old body back. It wasn't perfect, but it was familiar and it suited me just fine.

I used to think my legs were unattractive. Now I only remember how well they worked and wish I'd appreciated them before.

I want to fix myself, but the mirror is definitely not my friend today. The image looking back at me is that of a stranger, old and worn. She wears a look of undeniable fatigue. A little makeup would help and my hair is sticking up all funny, but at the moment I'm more hungry than I am concerned about my appearance.

My slippers make a swishing sound on the hardwood floor as I slide toward the kitchen. "Pick up your feet when you walk!" My mother's admonishment echoes back from childhood, but back then it was within my power to pick up my feet. Sorry, Mom. It's not my fault.

We have an average sized kitchen, a little on the old fashioned side, but it appears enormous to me now. A quick glance around and I take the easiest path to filling my belly, a slice of bread with peanut butter, and aim for the sofa. That's enough hard labor for now. Laying here and chatting with my mother on the phone, I find that it is becoming too difficult to hold the phone to my ear. I switch arms again and again until I can take it no more. "I have to hang up now, Mom. My arms hurt and I need a nap." My arms hurt from holding a phone to my ear? It sounds so ridiculous, even to me, that I wonder if she thinks I'm just blowing her off. That's what I would think if someone told me that.

The fatigue is winning again. It's more than just feeling tired. My whole body, brain and all, is wrapped up in this thick fog, stealing my personality and my ability to remain awake. I try channel surfing but, quite amazingly, the remote control is too much work. Yes, it's actually too tiring to change channels. I might be inclined to panic if I had the energy. It's hard to wrap my brain around this new development, but it doesn't matter because sleep overtakes me again.

Returning from errands later that week, Jim finds me occupying the exact same spot as when he left. "Glad you're home," says the slug.

He cautiously presents the cane he bought to help me move around a bit better. It's an ugly metal thing that reminds me of a nursing home or hospital, but what the heck, I'm willing to try. I think my grandmother used one like this before she graduated to a walker. But she wasn't still in her 40's at the time. I've aged several decades in the last six months. Jim tells me that choices were limited in the store but if I find it helpful, I should consider buying a nice cane.

He's right, of course. Obviously, MS isn't going to cut me any slack, so I'd better prepare for battle. We work on my form and when I hit the proper rhythm, the cane turns out to be very useful. It helps to keep me on an even keel rather than swaying and running off course, and I can lean on it a bit when standing still.

A few days later, while browsing some specialty cane sites online, I showed some of my choices to Jim. "I'm looking for something that doesn't jump out at you ... something that won't be particularly noticeable." It is typical of me, this effort to fade into the wallpaper, but he would have none of that.

Jim looked at me as though I'd lost my mind. "Are you kidding me? If you're going to use a cane, then USE A CANE!" The suggestion that bold is better makes sense. No wonder I love this man. Instead of being embarrassed by me and my cane, he is encouraging it. He wants what is best for me.

Okay, I will buy a cane and I will take ownership. I will use it with pride and dignity. I can almost hear the music swell. I will not fade quietly into the background because I need a little help. Look at me! I have a cane! A brightly colored paisley cane catches my eye. Red, blue, and gold, this adjustable cane also folds up, making it ideal for times when you are not sure you will need it. This thing has it all, so red paisley it is. For a fade-into-the-wallpaper gal like me, it is an interesting choice.

While we're at it, we decide to think about what else could help me when I'm relapsing. I've been having a lot of trouble in the kitchen. It turns out that standing still is even more taxing than walking. My legs want to fold under me and I end up having to brace myself against the kitchen counter as I work. That makes it hard to prepare food. We order a tall kitchen stool so that I can sit at a comfortable height when preparing dinner or doing the dishes.

Let's see, what else ... the shower has also been a trouble spot, so we add a shower chair to our order. This pro-active stance feels good. It's not about giving in; it's about discovering ways to remain active and productive. I don't have to rely on these things all the time, but it would be foolish to let pride get in the way when I do.

What bothers me most is not in the physical realm. It's what's going on inside my head that plagues me. What am I going to do now? I'm a useless blob half the time, aimlessly watching television and attempting to lose myself in books, succeeding only in becoming sleepier. I just spent 20 minutes staring at the painting on our living room wall. It's a beautiful painting, but I'm not really focusing on its beauty. I'm just staring, as though in a state of hypnosis. I'm beyond bored, but I have no idea how to manage this aspect of the new me. In fact, I'm tired of new me, but old me is missing in action.

Not so long ago, Jim and I regularly engaged in spirited conversation on a wide variety of topics, but now it seems all we talk about is MS. I suppose that's natural because we're still in the learning phase, but what else do I have to contribute? I can't do much and I have no sense of direction. I don't have a lot to offer Jim anymore.

Sleep seems to be my only relief from this train of thought.

CHAPTER 5
A Whole Other Level of "Stranger Danger"

The blob routine repeats itself for several more days before signs of recovery begin. Every day I am stronger and gaining dominion over my limbs.

Somehow I manage to get dinner on the table every night and consider this a small victory. I make a promise to myself that no matter what shape I'm in, no matter how little I may accomplish in a single day, I will reserve the energy necessary to prepare dinner, however simple. It's good to have goals.

After 10 days, I'm finally ready to attempt work again. Jim is going to have to drive me because I still can't completely trust my legs and arms to do what I tell them. I'm also using my new cane in public for the first time. I feel very conspicuous and self-conscious about it but, short of staying home forever, I don't have any choice.

Jim lets me out of the Subaru at the side entrance of the funeral home. The building itself seems to have grown in square footage since I was here last. I kiss Jim goodbye, sling my purse over my right shoulder, and grab the cane in my left hand.

I head toward the door, the cane making a slight clacking sound as it hits the pavement, reminding me of a nursing home again. With one hand on the door, I turn back and give Jim a nervous nod. I wonder what runs through his mind as he watches me walk away with the cane. I'm hardly the woman he fell in love with just a short time ago. As I pull the door open, I feel like the new kid on the first day of school.

They're surprised to see me, but I am welcomed back and complimented on my new paisley appendage. A few good-natured jokes later, I can let out a sigh of relief. I did it. I showed up in public using the cane and the earth did not alter its rotation.

Tom, one of the funeral directors, manages to find a path to humor in just about any situation. He's in a very somber line of work and is married to a woman with a serious autoimmune disease, so he's more than qualified to poke fun at life. He's an old pro at on-again off-again illness, and knows exactly the right attitude to take. He offers common ground and plenty of humor. I search his eyes for signs of pity, but find none. Maybe this won't be so bad after all.

My cane has a straight handle and no strap, so I can't hang it on anything. It folds up, but I don't want to have to fold and unfold every time I need to get up. I lean it against the wall and it slides and crashes on the floor. I pick it up and a few minutes later, it slides down again. Oh well, leave it there, then. I make a mental note to get a strap so I can at least get it off the floor and not have to worry about creating a booby trap.

The first time I need to use the restroom, I lean the cane against the stall while using the facilities. Now I am faced with a practical problem.

If I use the cane to get to the sink to wash my hands, if I don't also wash the cane handle, the whole procedure is moot. I begin a washing frenzy that seems without end, and soon I'm left feeling ridiculous and compulsive. But we are talking about the bathroom here. It's the little things.

In time, I will discover the horrors of being in the throes of a relapse and using a public restroom with hand blowers and no paper towels. Oh, that germ-ridden cane handle! It sounds like a trivial matter, and perhaps it is, but I need to avoid unnecessary illness. Things are difficult enough.

At this point, I can't even imagine what it would be like to try to navigate my world with a wheelchair. It's amazing how quickly our perceptions about the world can change.

A stranger in the halls of the funeral home stops me in my tracks. "Don't worry about your leg. I had to use a cane for a month, but it will heal. Just don't let yourself depend on that cane too much. Trust me." I smile and thank him before continuing on my way. He felt good about what he surely believed were comforting words, but I am stunned practically speechless by his presumptuousness. Because this is a funeral home, I tell myself he's probably grieving and was not thinking clearly about what he said. I didn't realize it on that day, but that was only my first taste of the type of incident that people with MS experience on a regular basis.

There will be an endless stream of unsolicited advice and commentary on my health and my attitude. Some of it will be heartfelt, some will cause me to scratch my head in wonder, some will hurt. It's a whole other level of "stranger danger."

It will happen on the street, at work, and at social events. I will be told – not asked – about my own health status based on how I happen to look in a single moment in time. Apparently, if I am able to sit in a chair and smile, I am in robust health. It's not that I resent being told I look good – it is the conjecture that goes along with it that I find offensive.

I will be given, in no uncertain terms, the cause and the cure for MS – dozens of them, from people who are convinced that their own remission equals a cure, heard it from a friend, or are just good old-fashioned con artists trying to take advantage. They all seem so certain in their assertions.

I will hear tales of great-aunt whoever, who suffered horribly and died a tragically premature death due to MS; and of cousin what's-his-name, who simply decided not to let it bother him, adopted a positive attitude, and became a super athlete and captain of industry.

Why do people assume that I haven't thought about and researched issues having to do with MS? Why do folks who've just met me think they have to explain it to me? Is this all anyone sees when they look at me anymore? I am capable of talking about other things.

Once, someone even introduced me by saying, "This is Ann. She has MS." Unfortunately, my quick retort and snappy comeback skills are seriously lacking. I've got to work on that.

Then there are the wise guys who think I don't have to worry about medical expenses because they mistakenly assume that I'm on Medicare. What? "Well, you're disabled." Really? It isn't as though you go to the doctor's office and come away with a diagnosis and Medicare card. And I do still work. The cold hard truth is that you have to be unable to work and you have to apply for and be accepted for Social Security Disability, which is not easy when you have an on-again, off-again invisible illness like MS. If and when you are accepted, you begin the two-year wait for Medicare eligibility. No, there is no easy button and I'm not on Medicare, not that it's anybody's business.

"MS may cause presumptuousness in others." This is something the medical journals should list under MS symptoms.

Then there is the opposite situation. Like the time we attended a crowded Christmas party and a woman carrying some glasses said, "Get the door for me, honey." I was leaning on the cane in my left hand, had a purse on my shoulder, and was balancing a wine glass in my right hand. Sheesh! The funny thing is, I managed to find a way to help her out. Score one for the MS lady! Those little victories are sweet tonic.

At 1:00 p.m. sharp, Jim pulls up to the side door and, although I am moving a lot slower than I was at 9:00 a.m., I am still moving. There's a lot to be said for that.

When we pull into the driveway at home, Jim grabs the mail. The bright blue handicapped placard has arrived. My doctor signed for a permanent one, so I'll never have to worry about getting a doctor's signature again.

Lucky me ... at least that's what people keep telling me, so why don't I feel lucky? Because this little placard is not a privilege. It is necessary if I am to avoid running out of steam before even reaching the entrance to a store or business. It will allow me to run errands by myself and hold on to precious remnants of independence. I tuck it away in the glove compartment and vow not to abuse it. Lucky indeed.

When speaking with someone with a disability or chronic illness, it is not a good idea to tell them they are lucky to have a handicapped-parking placard, even in jest. It is not a welcome trade for good health.

The same holds true of my work situation. Despite appearances that I have it easy, I don't consider myself fortunate to work half days. It is not a choice borne of privilege, but physical necessity. If luck has anything to do with it, it is most certainly not good luck. Work a half-day; get a half-day's pay and no benefits. Sounds like a dream. The little changes we've made these past few months give us a small measure of control over a situation that was growing frightfully out of control.

As the days pass, everything old is new again. I climb out of the depths of the latest attack, in a two-steps-forward, one-step-back kind of way. Finally, I am able to trust my driving skills again and put the cane away for the time being. Even the fatigue is granting sweet relief.

Maybe we can put this craziness behind us and concentrate on something else for a change. MS is taking up entirely too much of our lives, our thoughts, our conversations. Maybe this remission will last and maybe the medicine has had enough time to make a difference. We can't be all about MS. There's got to be more to us than that. We have to find a way to get back into real life again.

I'm sick to death of looking at the stack of videos and pamphlets that we received from the doctor, the pharmaceutical companies, and the National MS Society. It's all very informative and served its purpose, but I don't need to keep this stuff around anymore. We're swimming in it and it is becoming more of a hindrance than a help.

It all started with a seemingly benign but persistent tingly feeling in my right arm. We've come an awful long way since then. Back when my right leg first began to give me trouble, Jim was equally perplexed by the feelings I described and came up with an idea.

"Maybe your muscles are just achy. Let's try some BENGAY®." I'd never used BENGAY® before and had no idea what to expect.

"Let's just try it." Jim told me to sit and knelt on the floor in front of my leg.

"It's going to feel weird at first," he said as he rubbed a generous amount into the muscles of my thigh. Then he watched my face for reaction. Thirty seconds passed before he asked how it felt.

"I don't feel anything yet." The look on his face was of concern. We waited a few more minutes and the concern deepened.

"Don't tell me you can't feel that!"

"I don't feel anything. What should I be feeling?"

A few more minutes passed and he was getting anxious.

"Well, let's try another place. I'll put some on the back of your neck."

Within a minute I felt the intense cold/heat of the BENGAY® at work. Whoa!

Now I understood the look on Jim's face. It was the same look I observed in a neurologist's office when she performed the tuning fork test. Touching the fork to my foot, she instructed me to signal when I no longer felt the vibration. Upon my lack of response, Jim traded a quick glance with the doctor that spoke volumes. It's always awkward when people in the room trade "the glance" with each other but not with you. You never know where to look or how to react.

That seems so long ago now and all the educational material is cluttering up our home and cluttering up my mind. I step on tiptoes as I stretch to reach some videos on the bookshelf. I'm on my tiptoes! I haven't experienced this small pleasure for some time.

Smokey and Bandit follow my every move as I gather up the materials, haphazardly dumping them into a large trash bag and clumsily dragging it out of the house. I suddenly feel cleansed. I know I can't throw MS away, but I don't need to be reminded of it every waking moment.

It's hard to describe the feeling when the last remnants of an MS attack finally abate. It's like stepping back into my old body, my old self once again. I appreciate every step, every physical movement ... every emotion that makes me feel whole again.

I can't help but think about people who will never feel the high that comes with bouncing back from an attack. People who have progressive MS, spinal cord injury, or some other debilitating disease that never goes into remission, never get to feel this good again.

Relapsing/remitting MS puts me in a category of people who live a double life. One foot in the world of disability, one foot in the world of the able-bodied. We straddle both worlds, never fully belonging to either, alternating our physical reality on a daily basis. It's a mind-blowing way to live, but one in which the good days are keenly felt and appreciated. I am grateful for every movement, every stretch, every little glorious physical experience. Remission, though it may be temporary, is bliss.

CHAPTER 6
I Don't Want to be That Person

On Fourth of July weekend, Jim and I, along with my son Tommy, are taking a drive up to New Jersey to visit Jim's family. Jim's brother and his wife are hosting a holiday pool party for the family, and we've been looking forward to the weekend getaway and reconnecting with loved ones.

My MS is in a full remission and I feel strong and healthy. The cane is folded up in the back of the car, but I am sure I won't be needing it.

Tommy is in the back seat, looking comfortable with his earphones, and alternately lost in his tunes and nodding off. He doesn't like long car rides, but at least he's got his music.

Jim also appears to be lost in thought and I find myself glancing over in his direction often. I admire his half-smile and the curve of his arms as he gently guides the steering wheel. I know he's looking forward to spending time with family. He senses my prolonged gaze and laughs. "You're strange, you know that?"

"If it's strange to enjoy being with you then, yes, I'm strange."

He laughs again and rubs his arthritic right knee, which generally begins to ache after a few hours of highway driving.

Our relationship feels solid and secure. We are very much in love and, despite the health problems, we are closer than ever. Whatever the future holds, I know I've had more than my share of happiness.

This is nice. Jim and Tommy and me and a great weekend ahead with nary a thought of MS. Being with Jim's family will give us new things to talk about and, other than everyone asking how I'm doing at the outset, MS will likely play no part. Hallelujah!

The sun is bright and I put on my sunglasses, but something is not quite right. What *is* that? I instinctively close my eyes in the hope that I did not see what I think I saw.

No such luck. I see wavy lines out of the corner of my right eye, but when I try to focus on them, they move. Tricky little devils. Geometric patterns in shades of florescent green, deep red, and blackest black pop in and out. Tell me this is not happening. It's sort of like one of those creepy movie scenes where they are simulating a drug trip gone bad, and everything starts to bend and move. But I'm not on drugs, and this is not a movie.

In a few minutes, the wavy lines get weirder and start spreading toward the center of my field of vision. I'm beginning to get a little nervous, having read about visual disturbances – including blindness – in MS patients. How can it be that I'm sitting here with two other people, just inches away, who are oblivious to the fact that my world is now a psychedelic scene from a sixties movie?

I'm not going to say anything. I'm not going to say anything. This will stop in a minute.

I silently play games with the lines in an attempt to ignore the frightening possibilities. Try to look straight at them. Look away quickly. Still there. Close my eyes. Uh oh. Still there. The moving shapes and paint bucket of colors remain active, swirling and twirling and teasing. I'm not going to say anything.

Seconds turn to minutes. Minutes feel like hours. I am playing mind games with myself.

When it spreads to the left eye, I know it's time to let Jim in on what's happening over here in the passenger seat. When I turn toward him, there's a big hole where his right cheek should be. Oh, this can't be good. Am I about to go blind? I don't think I'll be handling that very well. Ridiculously inappropriate thoughts flood my brain – my eyebrows are a mess, who will keep them plucked for me ... how will I fix my hair and makeup ... I'll have to learn braille. Stop it!

"Sweetheart, uh ... I hate to tell you this, but something's wrong with my eyes." And there's that look again. I hate that look. It is a mixture of love and fear and responsibility and I don't know what, but it tears at my heart.

As I attempt to explain the inexplicable, the hole on his cheek keeps moving and I blink faster, thinking I can clear this whole thing up if I can just blink correctly and focus.

We don't want to alert Tommy to what is happening just yet, and luckily, he's still got the earphones on. The poor kid doesn't need this. Still, Jim's fear is palpable as he works at being the rock while keeping an eye on the road. I know what he's thinking. He's wondering what the hell he's going to do out here on the highway, on a holiday weekend, when I tell him I've gone blind.

I promise to keep him informed, but my emotions are fragile. I'm overwhelmed with intense anger at the situation. Here I am, strong again, finally holding my own, and my health has to take center stage again. I don't want to be that person – the one who always has a problem, the one who seems to be seeking attention at every turn. I just want to be me again. Imperfect, but intact, me. I don't want to be a drama queen and do not want to be the lead player in the "Persistent Perils of Poor Ann."

Blindness has always been a fear, but I try not to focus on that. Come on now and relax your mind. I'm kind of intrigued by the patterns and colors I see, and amazed that I can close my eyes and continue to see them. It's pretty awesome, actually. With that thought, I become consumed with guilt. What is wrong with me? How can I possibly find this interesting while Jim is probably having an internal freak out? How about that? Fear to anger to intrigue to guilt in just minutes. I could be my own Billy Mays infomercial.

"With the Amazing Ann you can turn emotions around on a dime! No more waiting for feelings to change! Order right now and we'll throw in an extra ounce of drama ..."

Within half an hour, vision in my right eye begins to return to normal. I announce the news to Jim and his relief is obvious. Ten minutes later, my left eye is normal as well. We've survived another crisis. I'm not blind. In fact, my vision is back to normal. Well, normal for me anyway. That was one of the strangest half hours of my life, and now it's over as quickly as it began. Who's going to believe this one?

Jim wants me to make an appointment with the neurologist first chance I get and I agree, but I know what that means. It means tests. If I've learned anything this past year it is that "tests" is a code word for torture. It means I will spend inordinate amounts of time in voice mail systems where none of the options is the correct one. I will leave messages that are never returned. My tests will be scheduled for three months from now. Someone will forget what room they put me in or why. The insurance company will provide a list of reasons why they won't pay. The price will be steep. It will be almost impossible to get someone to give me the results. The results will be inconclusive.

The wisdom in MS circles is that stress triggers exacerbations. Reducing stress is supposed to be crucial. I, however, am experiencing increasing levels of stress – not so much because I have this disease, not because of the symptoms and the limits it places on me, but because of my experiences dealing with the front office gauntlets of doctors' offices, medical insurance rules, and the financial impact this will have on our lives. How many forms have I filled out in the past year, how many inquiries, how many hours spent on the red tape that goes along with medical care and insurance? Too many. But I will attempt the obstacle course anyway because it's all we've got to work with.

My mind wanders back a few months. I was resting on the flat table and checking my watch again for perhaps the dozenth time. I could have died by now and no one would know. There's no call button and no one has bothered checking on me, not even once. Funny, when they gave me the spinal tap, they told me that I should not be left alone and that I should not stand up for a full hour. They said they would bring Jim in to stay with me during this crucial time. I hear voices in the hallway, but no one enters the room. It's been an hour and fifteen minutes now and I can't stop thinking about how worried Jim must be. I decide to get up anyway and open the door. Someone from a group of health care workers – I don't know if they are doctors, nurses, or what, because they all dress the same these days – looks at me and says, "Hey, you're not supposed to be up!" Great. At least I finally got their attention. They had simply forgotten about me.

Tommy unplugs and asks what we're talking about, but is unfazed by our explanation. Upon hearing that I'm really quite well, he returns to his music and we close in on New Jersey, where we will celebrate Independence Day with family, lounge around the pool, and feast on fine Italian food.

For the next few days, at least, I appear to all to be the very picture of health. That is the beauty and the curse of MS.

Ann Pietrangelo

CHAPTER 7
Pointing Out the Obvious

"Look what I can do!" It's a quote from an old skit on *Mad TV* about a goofy and completely untalented and uncoordinated kid named Stuart, who follows that line with an awkward hop and expectations of high praise from bored observers.

A couple of my co-workers are also familiar with Stuart, so I use the line whenever I want to show them how well I'm doing. Today, "Look what I can do!" is followed by a few skips and a jump down the hall of the funeral home; probably not something you see every day.

They laugh along with me – I'm pretty sure it's not at me – and applaud my strength, if not my grace.

The gang at work has a front row seat on my roller coaster ride through the world of relapsing/remitting multiple sclerosis, and I don't mind the audience.

Recently, I made what seemed like a thousand-mile trek to the front reception desk. Pausing to make small talk, my legs began to get that "uh oh" kind of feeling. In one of those all too predictably unpredictable MS moments, my legs turned to Jello™.

I leaned back against the wall, but I was still losing ground. Unable to fight gravity, I let myself slip down the wall until I hit the bottom ... or should I say until my bottom hit ... hoping nobody would wander by to witness my miscalculation. MS is not concerned about appearances. That's something you learn early on. If you're going to worry about strange looks, you're in for a rough time.

Since I was down there anyway, I stretched my legs straight out and rested for a moment. In complete denial of my situation, I continued chatting away as if there were nothing amiss. Who'll notice? Suddenly realizing how this might look and not wanting to create a scene should an unsuspecting member of the public arrive, I decided I'd better get back on my feet. Trying to be nonchalant about the whole thing, I braced myself between my cane and the wall in an effort to force my body up, while still carrying on a conversation. With legs splayed, I awkwardly rocked myself back up and onto my feet.

Several people happened by just in time to catch me in the act and rushed over to save me from myself. "And that," I said, "is why I never wear dresses!" Laughs all around.

Depleted of energy by then, I grabbed a chair to rest for a moment. Tom, recognizing the signs of MS run amok, seized on the opportunity to make a full-out production of my predicament, even while lending a hand. With an exaggerated flourish, he grabbed the back of my chair and pushed me – chair and all – through the hallways, to my office, and right up to my desk, waving at passersby and laughing all the way. Good thing there wasn't a funeral going on.

Every now and then, someone presents me with a new cane for my growing collection. I now have a very lightweight bamboo cane, a cane with a brass duck head, and one with a silver elephant head.

When using a cane in public, I attract a certain amount of attention, probably because I look too young, or because I look as though I don't really need one. That's the thing about the cane. If I use correctly, it does appear that I don't need it. I like that, but it's confusing to strangers, who often approach me to make small talk about it. Some stare outright, but some folks are concerned and genuinely want to know what's wrong. I've been saying stupid things like, "I just have weak legs," or "my legs need a little help," in an attempt to deflect their questions. After months of listening to this, Jim points out the obvious.

"What are you doing? Why don't you just say you have MS? It's the truth and there's nothing wrong with that." He's right, of course. I have no acceptable answer to his question. It's just been a subtle and subconscious avoidance of the issue. Not that strangers have any right to my private health status, but I need not shy away from the truth. It's what I have, not who I am. I have MS. It rolls off the tongue easily enough now when I am among friends, so why not take the leap altogether? From now on, "I have MS" will be my answer. Maybe I can even enlighten a few folks along the way.

When I'm strong and healthy things are every bit as askew as they are when I'm relapsing. I feel strange and out of sync either way. By the time I get used to the disabilities, I'm better again. It happens so slowly that I have to remind myself, "Oh, yeah! I can go for a long walk now."

As soon as I start to feel secure and on sure-footing, those warning signs appear and remind me that my able-bodied freedom will not last. Time to get in all those errands I'd like to run by myself.

"It's complicated." I've heard people use that phrase to describe a relationship, and it's a good way to describe my relationship with MS. I have disabilities ... yet I don't. It is unclear to which, if either, world I belong. I fight being labeled even as I simultaneously search for the proper label.

Who I am and how I relate to the world around me is in a never-ending state of flux and I have no way of knowing when and where I will settle in, if ever. I'm beginning to understand the truth – that change will be the constant in my world, and if I can embrace that philosophy, I'll be okay. Change is the constant in everyone else's world, too, but there are certain times in our lives when we settle in and allow ourselves to believe that this is how things will always be. I don't believe I'll ever make that mistake again.

I'm seriously questioning what I'm doing with my life. Do I really need to limit myself to part-time work? Shouldn't I be doing more? I'm feeling woefully inadequate, questioning myself and my abilities. Am I really trying hard enough? Is it the MS that sparks all the questions, or my age?

Maybe it's my 45th birthday that's gotten to me. It's a fact that I'm a middle-aged woman. I struggle with that thought, but the numbers don't lie. I'm too young to call it a day and retire. I'm too old to start wondering what I want to be when I grow up, but that's precisely what I'm doing. I have to figure out how I can remove my physical self from that thought process.

MS is often diagnosed in people who are in their forties, and that's already a somewhat tumultuous decade, at least it is for me. Major life changes, from divorce to relocation have already stirred the pot. I miss my family; I miss my kids. I miss having a "real" job. MS simply adds to the insecurities and doubts that swirl around inside my head.

There's a lot of talk these days about people reaching middle-age and redefining themselves, both personally and professionally, and this is exactly what I must do. It is irrelevant whether I came to this point by force or of my own free will.

The thing is, I've never really had a career. I've had a variety of jobs, some better than others. My first stab at employment was as a nurses' aid in a nursing home, helping to feed and bathe elderly bedridden patients. It was extremely physical work and at some other point in my life would have been very gratifying, but at 16-years-old, I was emotionally unprepared for the heartache that came with it. I lasted all of six months.

Later, while still in high school, I applied for a job on an assembly line at a local factory. It was literally just a few steps from my own front door, so the location was ideal. My hometown, Woonsocket, Rhode Island, was built on factories and factory labor. A large percentage of the previous generation, blue collar or white, spent a big chunk of their working years in one factory or another. My oldest brother and sister had already done time on the line, so I had some idea what to expect.

The factory manufactured Christmas ornaments and my job title was "clipper." So what exactly does a Christmas ornament clipper do?

We clippers were to attach the little circular wire thing, the one used to hook the ornaments to the tree, to the top of the ornaments as they rolled past us. If there is a name for that little doohickey, I don't know what it is, but for awhile it was a very important part of my day. This was on-your-feet, toe-the-line sweaty mill work, and we had to do so many clips per minute in order to fill the boxes before they reached the end of the line.

The first day on the job was the toughest. They brought most of us right in and put us on the line. They explained that you had to do so many clips per minute ... or else. Out came the stopwatch. Shortly after that, the dismissals began. I'm proud to say I was a pretty fast clipper, although it's not something I would include on a resume.

There was a certain amount of pressure to keep up. If the clippers don't fill the boxes before they get to the end of the line, the resulting backup makes for angry supervisors and a very unpleasant day. Think Lucy in the chocolate factory. It was on this job that I developed a keen appreciation for hard but honest work, an education in teamwork, and a good idea of how I didn't want to spend my life.

There are things I learned on the line that have stayed with me through the years, with the added benefit of having a great odd job story. I once sat around a dinner table where discussion turned to weird jobs. I was unanimously voted the winner.

From there I graduated to nice office jobs, each one better than the last, finally settling in with trade associations, work I thoroughly enjoyed. There's a certain rush in working toward a trade show or convention for months and finally seeing it all come together.

Then came a 12-year stint raising three children full-time — easily the most challenging and rewarding work there is. After that, it was like starting over again, going from part-time office work and back into association work, before MS derailed all that.

Just prior to my current job at the funeral home, I was working at a trade association located 60 miles from home. The hour and fifteen minute one-way commute proved to be too much for my legs and arms to bear. Even though I had yet to receive a diagnosis, I had little choice but to look for work closer to home. I'd barely settled in at that job before having to resign.

So where do I go from here? I didn't have a plan in high school and I certainly don't have a plan now. I still haven't figured out what I want to be when I grow up! It took MS to make me actually attempt to answer that question.

Well, I'm all grown up now, and I have to evaluate my strengths and weaknesses; I must balance the physical with the intellectual, and throw in a dash of emotion.

There's no doubt that a similar balancing act is going on in Jim's inner sanctum. This isn't exactly what he bargained for either. I leave him a wide berth for his thought process, confident that he will work it out in his very analytical, yet very heartfelt way, and that I will be able to accept his conclusions in a dignified manner. I hope we survive this together because I am hopelessly, outrageously, teenagerishly in love. There is a small speck somewhere in my heart that is preparing for the possibility that we will crash and burn because MS just might be a game-changer.

MS varies greatly from person to person, ranging from complete disability to being barely a blip on the radar. Nevertheless, my doctor has said that my case is unusual. Relapsing/remitting MS doesn't normally manifest itself in this manner.

My exacerbations come at almost perfect intervals, presenting with the same symptoms in the same order and then reversing the process. Part of the deal with relapsing/remitting MS is the mind games it plays with you. Guilt and self-doubt plague its unwilling hosts, and I'm no exception.

I spend a lot of time wondering if I should ... if I could ... do more. I worry about how other people perceive me. Do they think I'm faking, or making excuses ... do they think the cane is a prop ... do they make snide remarks about my handicapped-parking placard?

I'm starting to hear a lot about the power of positive thinking and pushing oneself to the limits, and I wonder what people are really trying to say. Do they think I relapse because of a bad attitude? I think Jim would agree that I have a fine attitude, but the relapses come anyway.

Some days my efforts are no less than herculean; something I'm not sure even Jim realizes. Simply getting through my day doing what I need to do is quite an accomplishment, but you wouldn't know it to look at me. I'm doing the best I can, but I feel as though I'm supposed to climb mountains and run marathons to prove that I've got my attitude on straight. But who, exactly, am I trying to impress?

Worrying about what other people perceive to be the truth is a pointless waste of time and energy – two things I can no longer squander. It is time to cast away some of those childlike insecurities.

I wouldn't choose to have a chronic disease like MS as a teacher, but it seems the lessons have begun anyway.

CHAPTER 8
No More Secs!

It is Christmas Eve and for the first time this year, all three of my kids are here together. I'm starting to feel the warning signs of imminent relapse, but am determined to make it through the next week without too much trouble. I can't let MS interfere with our time together.

Because of the long trip from the airport right at dinnertime, I had to do most of the prep work for dinner beforehand. Our unusual Christmas Eve dinner consists of spaghetti, home made tomato sauce, and Italian sausage and peppers, all liberally seasoned with garlic. They are understandably ravenous after their trip and eager to dig in. I'm just so happy to have everyone together that we could be eating peanut butter and jelly and it would feel like a gourmet meal.

After dinner we present David with a belated birthday gift – his birthday was last week – and indulge in a cake I made from a mix. He tends to shy away from the whole birthday thing, so we skip the candles and the song. We bought him a much-needed set of luggage, a not so subtle hint that we'd like him to visit more often.

I'm having a bit of an adrenaline rush from the excitement, so I stay up until the wee hours of the morning, talking and laughing with them long after Jim retires for the night. He didn't say so, but I know darn well he did that to give me some time alone with them. It's very typical of him.

We reminisce about their early childhood, as we are prone to do, laughing at the silly things they did, and my sometimes unintentionally offbeat response.

"Remember the time we all ...?"

"Remember when you said …?" On and on we reminisce, interrupting each other in our quest for laughs. When they were little tykes, we would dance like fools to the tune of Billy Joel's "Pressure" as a prelude to chores. Unconventional perhaps, but it sure got them moving. Those goofy little things have a tendency to stick in the mind.

One of our favorite stories is the evening I was calling for the kids to come to the dinner table. Liz and Tommy came to the table quickly, but David said, "Just a sec." He was completely wrapped up in a video game, so I allowed time for him to complete the level or whatever the heck he needed to do in order to pause. The trouble is that parents and children live in different time zones.

A few minutes later I called him again, "Come on, David, it's time for dinner!"

"One sec" came the reply again.

Now I'm a patient woman, but after three or four more cries of, "One sec!" I lost my cool, and in my best authoritative mom voice called out, "No more secs!"

A stunned silence followed, then a burst of laughter at my ill-chosen reprimand. "Mom said no more sex! Mom said no more sex!" They sang my words over and over, pointing at me, giggling uncontrollably and dancing around until I joined them in laughter. I'd already lost my authority anyway.

It's one of those lines that in time becomes part of family lore, brought up again and again at each gathering, getting even funnier as the years pass. "Remember the time Mom told us no more sex?" Oh, I'll never live that one down.

We awoke on Christmas morning with all three of my kids under the same roof. I couldn't ask for a better gift; I was beside myself with joy. Jim made a wonderful meal of eggs and ham and we lingered at the breakfast table, placing calls to his daughters and his parents, then to my mother.

Our Christmas tree is, well, a bit different. It's only four feet high, but we decorate it with plenty of colorful lights and assorted ornaments and it is quite lovely. It sits atop an unusual side table with the "see no evil, hear no evil, speak no evil" monkeys under a glass top. We purchased it on a whim even though we really had no use for it other than as a conversation piece. Cute as it is, the monkeys don't exactly go with the holiday motif, so I cover the table with a decorative Christmas tablecloth. Unfortunately, the tablecloth is not quite long enough to cover them completely, so the monkeys' feet stick out from the bottom. Brightly wrapped gifts hide them now, but soon they'll be showing again, creating a bizarre little display of a Christmas tree with monkey feet. I always have the best of intentions to remedy this oddity, but somehow I never get around to it. We don't set out to be contrary; it seems to come naturally.

We turn on the Christmas lights and cue the seasonal music. Gathering in the living room, the kids present their gift first.

They bought us yet another set of wine glasses, setting off a round of good-natured giggling. It has become a running joke that we need a new set every year because we somehow manage to break the glasses on a regular basis. I don't know what it is about wine glasses, but we – both of us – do manage to break a lot of them. There shall be no expensive crystal for us.

The kids unwrap their gifts and it's hugs all around. Christmas is missing something when there are no little kids around to make a mess with all the wrappings or tear up the house with new toys. I mentioned that to Jim awhile ago, so he indulged me with a box of Crayolas™, one tub of blue Play-Doh™ (ah, the aroma of Play-Doh™), and an Etch-a-Sketch™, one of my favorite childhood toys. There is no age limit on an Etch-a-Sketch™ and everyone wants a turn. I plan to pull them out every year with the holiday decorations and place them around the tree, just for that old-time Christmas feeling. Maybe we should add a Slinky™. A little nostalgia goes a long way.

Tommy spends the afternoon downstairs watching a new wrestling DVD we just gave him. He has an intense interest in professional wrestling and is studying the moves. David is catching up on some much-needed sleep and Jim is relaxing in front of the TV.

Liz keeps me company in the kitchen as I prepare Christmas dinner – glazed ham, sesame green beans, sweet potato fries, green salad, and bread fresh from the bread machine, followed by some angel food cake with fresh strawberries.

We set a lovely table in the dining room and light some candles. Conversation is bubbly and I'm thoroughly enjoying having the people I love most breaking bread around the same table at the same time. I want this meal to last forever, but eventually we've had our fill.

Everyone pitches in to clear the table and put away the leftovers. That ham is going to be even better tomorrow. Jim, Tommy, and Liz scatter to enjoy a post-dinner slump. David takes the initiative and starts washing dishes, while I wipe. We use the time for some one-on-one conversation. I greatly cherish these moments. All at once I can see my little babies underfoot, hanging on my legs and the young adults they have become. I can't help but think the world is a better place with them in it.

I'm beginning to feel tired again. It was bound to happen. Yesterday's adrenaline rush couldn't last forever, and I've really been pushing it today. I think I can hide it for awhile. I don't want to miss a single minute of this visit.

A couple of hours later we meet at the television and settle in to watch one of the movies the kids brought with them. But first we've got to make some popcorn. Jim takes out the sturdy old pan, blackened with years of dripping oil, and places it on the stovetop. It is truly the ugliest pan in America, but we wouldn't part with it for anything. I take out the popcorn seeds, canola oil, and five suitably large bowls.

Jim has taken over the main task of popping corn, and he does so with a certain amount of what I will loosely refer to as "flair." He always overfills the pan with seeds, which then push up forcefully against the cover. He pours the top layer of popcorn into a bowl before placing it back on the stove. He generally loses a handful of popcorn and a smattering of unpopped seeds in the process. It is a delightful mess and he puts me in mind of an overworked short order cook. It is quite an enjoyable little performance. Butter, salt, drinks ... we're ready to settle in. Ah, this is the life.

While everyone else is engrossed in the movie, I'm trying to savor the moment and burn it into my consciousness so that I may carry it with me always. I wish for time to stand still, freezing us forever in our little cocoon world, but I know that's not a fair wish. These kids – young adults – have no such desire. They are at an age of impatience and a longing for bigger and better things ... and rightly so.

The holidays conclude with my tears in the airport terminal. The trio always looks at me as though I've become unhinged, but none of them has ever been a mother.

Physically, the last few days have been more difficult than I wanted to admit. I never do as good a job with hiding it as I think, and Jim always knows anyway, even if he doesn't mention it. He observes the little missteps, the widening gait, the slumping posture that foretell the coming battle. Maybe it's really me that I'm trying to fool.

We were largely spared for the holidays, but it is apparent that we are wanted in the ring for another round. The weight of this realization is compounded by my post-holiday, post-kid visit letdown.

I've got the blues ... I'm going to have to get a handle on this thing.

CHAPTER 9
It Depends On What You Mean by Inconspicuous

The doctor ordered another round of steroids and I'm going out of my mind with this stuff. I fail to see the benefit of the last round, but agreed to give it another try anyway. It's going to take a while to figure out how we're going to approach MS for the long term, but for now I am imprisoned in a vicious cycle.

It is day four of the dreaded drip and the usual room is closed on Saturday, so they sent me to another floor of the hospital where confusion reigns supreme. Nobody seems to know why I'm here, where my meds are, or who is supposed to administer them.

"What is this for again?"

"Who authorized it?"

"Where's the order?"

They stuck me in a lonely room by myself while they are supposedly sorting it all out. I repeatedly walk down the hall to remind them of my existence, but there seems to be different personnel in charge every time. It's a good thing my life doesn't depend on this drip.

The 90-minute drip tied me up for six hours and, even though I was polite and smiling through it all, I am beside myself with frustration. Back at home, Jim is too, thinking I've disappeared forever inside the hospital maze.

Please tell me this is not going to be my life now — intravenous drips and hospitals, trapped in an endless cycle of tests and re-tests and repetitive nonsense. I am rapidly losing any semblance of control I might once have felt. I do not want to be a professional patient. I do not want to spend the rest of my life at the mercy of MS. So far, I've been doing what I'm told to do, not effectively or thoroughly questioning all options, and getting little guidance from the medical community. I feel like the ball in a pinball machine, bouncing haplessly from bumper to bumper at the mercy of an unseen player.

It's obvious that something is going to have to change. Maybe I don't need so much intervention and intrusion in my life. It could just be that it exacerbates the situation more than it helps.

And now, ladies and gentlemen, a big round of applause ... please welcome Mania back to the show!

Part of me is thrilled to be pumped with energy to burn for a change. The killjoy part of me knows that I'll pay the price eventually. Whether or not the treatment is good for my MS in the long run is not easy to assess, even for the doctors. So many things about MS fall into the gray zone and it's all but impossible for anyone, even a neurologist, to tell you what the right course of action should be. There are no cut and dry answers, and we patients have to work our way through it, trying to meld medical science with the reality of our own lives. This is no simple task, and one that calls for constant reevaluation.

If I could only manage to shut up for a few minutes, it might not be so unbearable. I seriously dislike being me right now. The good news is that I'm running around like gangbusters again, a super hero in action. The bad news is that I can't focus on what it is I should be doing, flitting from one task to another and in the end accomplishing little. But the flurry of activity makes me feel young and alive again. There's something to be said for that.

I can't sleep and can't keep my eyes closed, creating an endless stream of thought that, if left unchecked, will surely drive me mad. My brain is in overdrive, even at night, in an endless circle of contemplation – *the bathroom needs cleaning, we should take that ratty kitchen wallpaper down, what's Liz up to, I really could work full days, is Jim sorry he ever met me, what's going to become of me, any good movies on?*

The wavy eye thing is coming and going again, but we've since learned that this is caused by ocular migraines – migraines without pain and most likely unrelated to MS. It's a bizarre new twist, but we're told that it is nothing to be concerned about, so we add it to our growing list of things to get used to. Rolling with the punches is becoming second nature.

So that kitchen wallpaper is really getting to me. It's old, probably put up in the 70's, from the looks of it, and years of sunlight and kitchen grease give it a listless appearance. It looks depressing and I don't think I can stand it another minute. No, I really can't.

In a moment of heightened awareness and energy, I decide to do something about it. I pull and wiggle the stove until there is enough space for me to squeeze behind it. Look at me moving a stove! Oh, yeah, that's right, I'm bad. Nothing can stop me now.

Locating an inconspicuous spot to ascertain how difficult the job would be, I begin to peel away at a seam. Obviously, the previous homeowners intended this wallpaper to last until the year 2050 and if I don't interfere, it probably will. It is secured to the wall within an inch of its life and there is a border plastered over it at the top and at the bottom.

Despite my lack of a plan or proper tools, and without the slightest consideration of how I might feel about the job five minutes from now, I start pulling tiny pieces away and moving higher and higher up the wall.

What have I done? I am now committed to an enormous project. Did I mean to do this? Oh, well. It's kind of fun.

After work the next day I assemble supplies and go at it again, driven by steroids and an overwhelming need to accomplish something tangible. The work is hard, especially in the upper corners of the room, but I press on, dropping tiny shreds of sticky wallpaper all over the floor, countertops, appliances, and myself. Squirt bottles, scrapers, ladder, paint samples, dishes to be washed ... it looks like a disaster struck this room, but I am quite determined, and for several days am completely consumed by the process.

I wrangle Jim into coming to the hardware store with me to pick out a paint color. What must he be thinking, as I dismantle our kitchen and pretend to know what I am doing? He's either very happy that I'm doing a chore he is not interested in tackling himself, or he's just relieved that I have something to focus on, sparing him endless chatter. Or maybe he's giving it no thought whatsoever.

A few more days on the job and my cyclone of energy is beginning to unravel. The kitchen is a mess and it's obvious that I'm spinning toward a powerful relapse. I'm having trouble lifting my arms up high enough and it's starting to hurt.

Jim senses the crash coming from miles away and rescues me by painting the edges and the ceiling line while I roll paint on the final wall. Every last ounce of strength drains from me as Jim collects the used materials and gets the kitchen back to working order. We are quite pleased with the outcome and I can take pleasure in the knowledge that I have accomplished something. The kitchen looks great! No matter what happens in the weeks to come, I can always look at the kitchen walls with a feeling of satisfaction for a job well done.

I'm having trouble standing and walking. I've already given up driving again. On the morning that I can no longer hold the blow dryer up long enough to dry my hair, I know it's time to stop working, too. If I cannot blow dry my own hair, trying to function at work would be a serious mistake. That seems to be a fair predictor, one which I will continue to use as a gauge of my strength each morning.

I'm down for the count. Jim doesn't even bother waking me up for work, instead calling in for me and letting me sleep. He is amazed at how many hours I can sleep and still be tired, but he knows it is beyond my control. The doctor gave me some medication to fight the fatigue, but it acts in much the same manner as the steroids and prevents me from sleeping at all. It's not worth it. None of this seems worth it right now. I can't decide what's worse ... MS or the plan to fight MS. Then again, there doesn't seem to be a plan. I think I know how lab rats feel.

I'm not at all the person I was last month, or the person I was last week. MS is unpredictable. I am unpredictable. I catch a glimpse of myself in the full-length mirror and cannot match the self-image in my mind with the reflection. Who is that person? Deplorable posture, messy hair, worn look. If I had the strength, I'd cry.

The energetic stream of consciousness is eventually replaced by one continuous, sleepy, foggy mess of days and nights melting together with little sense of purpose. I am merely existing.

When I awake, it takes me awhile to locate all my limbs. Sometimes they are tingly, like after a limb falls asleep, but sometimes I don't feel them at all, as though they were detached from my body.

I want to, but I never quite get to a bona fide out-of-body experience. To give up the weighty vessel that carries us must be very freeing.

I dangle my feet on the floor to test the waters. How bad is it going to be today? Can I feel my toes? Will I be able to move more than a few steps? Then to the shower and the daily attempt at a beauty routine. My wardrobe these days consists mostly of a robe and slippers. Eat. Nap. Watch mindless television. Try to focus brain on something productive. Shuffle around house. Attempt to appear human. Read until drowsy, a process that takes all of 30 seconds these days.

I begin evaluating my energy levels around 3:00 p.m., thinking about what will be required to complete a presentable dinner in my freshly painted kitchen. I promised myself I would manage this task every day and I intend to stick to it. I put my feet up and try to mentally conjure up the right amount of energy. "Just get through dinner ... just get through dinner ..." It's all I have to do before I can collapse.

Then it's time to rest again and lounge around until bedtime, which comes frighteningly early these days.

My world is getting smaller and smaller, until I'm sure I will cease to exist at all. I've memorized every square inch of the living room walls and know exactly how many baby steps it is from the sofa to the kitchen counter. Somewhere around step number nine it gets frustrating.

The baby steps put me in mind of *The Carol Burnett Show*, in which Tim Conway hilariously portrayed a shuffling old man character. The old guy with the wild white hair took forever to get across a room, taking almost imperceptible baby steps, while acting as though running like the wind. Audiences roared with laughter at his antics, and I can't help but smile at the memory now. It is amazing how television shows from the 70's manage to come back to me at the craziest of times. I suppose it's because I was a rather lonely teenager, so television was a big part of my life.

"How're you doin' babe?"

"I'm hanging in there." It is an effort to call back to him.

I try not to dwell on it, but I wonder how he is managing all this. I'm quite a sight and it's got to be disturbing as hell that I am so completely dependent upon him. For now, at least, I am quite disabled.

As supportive and loving as he is, surely he must question the wisdom of a long-term relationship with me. I know he loves me, but my MS is becoming a titanic problem, one that is changing everything about the relationship we thought we would have. Medicine may not work for me and with such frequent relapses, I fear the onset of a more progressive form of MS.

In the pattern that has become so familiar, I gain a little strength every day and gradually find myself again. The days begin to distinguish themselves from the nights by sheer routine. I can fix my hair and put on makeup. The robe and slippers are replaced by pants and blouses and shoes that feel heavier than I remembered. At last, I am ready to brave the working world again.

"Welcome back," Jim says to me as I manage to complete my morning routine for the first time in eight days. "I feel as though I lose you when you have that fatigue. You seem so far way."

Indeed, I was very far away. Far away from him, far away from me and everything I ever knew about myself.

It will still be weeks before I can get through the afternoon without a nap, put away the cane, or drive safely again. This is an emotionally exhausting stage of the game, the time when appearances are especially deceiving. Trust me, it's harder than it looks.

The MS relapses are stealing my personality. The sheer magnitude of the symptoms is all-consuming. I've got to do something about that.

I'm making another promise to myself – to find a way to stay in the game when in the throes of full-blown relapse. I cannot let myself simply slip away. The beast must be tamed.

Ann Pietrangelo

CHAPTER 10
I Would If You Asked

It's early February, one year since diagnosis, and we've lived through the extreme highs and lows of life with multiple sclerosis. It has been a tough year, but we've settled in to a comfortable routine.

It's just the two of us here, with Smokey and Bandit, and our home has a peaceful feel to it. We decorated in soothing colors and clean lines. Neither of us is a fan of clutter, so there is plenty of breathing room, except for our home office. The smallest room in the house is tightly packed, with two desks, two file cabinets, tons of books, and two Macs. Jim would sooner quit using computers altogether than allow a PC into the house. Just one of those techie-guy things. It's almost comical how often all four of us are crammed into this tiny room together. Guess we would manage well enough in a one-room cabin.

Jim has become so attuned to my physical state that it's downright spooky. He understands without asking why I tend to lean against him in public, or hold his hand or arm when we walk together.

He can sum up my gait in a matter of seconds, calculating my level of disability. He no longer asks me why I look so sad. He recognizes that look now as one of extreme fatigue, not sadness. Clearly, he doesn't like it, but he made his peace with my need for naps and frequent breaks.

Jim understands me and loves me for who I am. He knows that a fancy piece of jewelry given on the prescribed holiday holds little meaning compared to how he treats me every day. He looks me in the eye when he speaks and, better yet, he looks me in the eye when I speak. He treats me with respect and dignity. He engages in an emotional foreplay that lasts all day and can even manage to get through to me when MS has me on the ropes.

I like to think I do as much for him. He's the kind of guy who doesn't ask for or need much beyond love and respect and kindness, and I give him those in abundance. Every indication is that he appreciates that.

What makes it all work, I think, is that we like each other. It's easy enough to fall head over heels in love, but if you don't like each other – if you wouldn't be friends if you weren't lovers – love will eventually kick you in the butt.

We've become two parts of a single unit, seldom separated for more than a few hours. Despite the setback of MS, our life together is a good one. It is possible that illness has actually drawn us closer, forcing us to move more slowly, appreciating every step along the way.

Dinner has become the cherished ritual, the daily event that kicks off the evening. I usually serve in the kitchen, around 6:30 p.m. Neither of us is particularly fond of our beat up old kitchen table, but neither do we speak of replacing it. There is something strangely comforting about the old wooden clunker, and we don't mind the cats clawing at the rough underbelly.

We enjoy traveling and going out, but at heart we are a couple of homebodies and, left to our own devices, will favor staying home and watching a movie while enjoying a bowl of popcorn. Every now and then, we have to kick ourselves in the pants and force ourselves to go out, whereupon we generally have a good time.

The real danger in a relationship like ours is that we are so similar in our opinions and personalities that we constantly reinforce each other rather than give an opposing view. Fortunately, we both have a tendency to look at things from all angles and seek outside input.

I prepare simple, healthy dinners with generous helpings of fresh vegetables and salads. More often than not, I light candles and play music. No television or telephones allowed. It's a shame that so many families have given up on sharing the evening meal together. They are truly missing out.

The most important ingredient in the kitchen is tomato sauce, of that I have no doubt. It took some time, but I finally picked up on the fact that the way to Jim's stomach is through tomato sauce. If I run out of ideas, all I have to do is pour tomato sauce over – well, pretty much anything – and dinner will be a hit.

Thanks to Jim's mother, I finally learned how to make my own tomato sauce. She gave me the basics and I add a little extra zip of my own. I know I'll never match her kitchen skills or intimate knowledge of fine Italian cooking, but I'm not hearing any complaints on the home front, either.

Dessert is never part of the ritual, but a glass of wine usually is. Lately we've developed quite an interest in wine, attending tastings and visiting local vineyards. The Shenandoah Valley is home to some stunning scenery. There's a lot to be said for the serenity of lounging outdoors with a mountainous backdrop, a glass of wine, and the love of your life.

We recently purchased a small plaque that says, "In wine there is truth," hanging it in a prominent place over one of the kitchen entryways. Heaven knows I do have a tendency to speak more freely after a glass of wine.

Tonight I've got a Dean Martin CD playing while we eat baked tilapia, fresh brussels sprouts (a much maligned vegetable) with garlic, and green salad with no tomatoes. Despite his affection for all things with tomato sauce, Jim will not eat an actual tomato. I find that strangely endearing. In traditional European style, we eat the salad last.

We're both enjoying a glass of Pino Grigio. As usual, Jim lays his utensils across his plate long before I do, and lingers over the wine while I finish my meal.

Conversation is light and easy. I am in great physical shape, having fully bounced back from the latest attack, and I'm keenly aware of how fantastic I feel. Right now I am not disabled in the least, and I'm taking full advantage of that fact. I feel my age again. Jim is obviously enjoying the benefits of my remission as well. In a very brief period of time, MS has been relegated to the recent past.

Finally, we rise and begin to clear the table. Suddenly Jim stops, leaning against the stove, and pulls me closer, wrapping his arm loosely around my waist. "What would you say if I asked you to marry me?"

"Oh, I'd marry you if you asked," I laughed. We've danced around the topic of marriage before.

"I am asking. Will you marry me?"

He's wearing that lopsided grin of his, looking me straight in the eye, and it's clear that he is quite serious. The tears come quickly, streaking down my cheeks and making my voice crack.

"Yes!"

We kiss and hold each other tightly for a few moments, soaking in the moment. Right here, in our little kitchen, under the watchful eyes of Smokey and Bandit and amidst the dirty dinner dishes, a monumental life decision is made.

We're in our forties and we've both been down this road a time or two already. Actually, this is the third try for each of us. It's not something either of us is proud of, but something that must be acknowledged. We can only hope that a double-third is the charm, and we're wearing the goofy grins of teenagers in love for the first time. No words could adequately capture how much I love this man, or even how much I feel loved in return.

We've discussed the uncertainty of my health status ad infinitum this past year and there is nothing that needs to be said about it tonight. I know that Jim has given this a great deal of thought, mentally listed the pros and cons, and decided of his own free will to take his chances as my mate for life.

"Ann, you're in a good place right now – almost back to 100 percent – I think we should get married right away so we can enjoy the day and a honeymoon while you're strong. If we wait, we'll be taking a chance on another relapse spoiling it."

That's an excellent point. It warms my heart that he speaks about the probability of ill health to come, but only for planning purposes.

Of course I want to enjoy a week away with my new husband, but there's so much more to consider. We've got families – parents, siblings, and children spread around the country. Most haven't even met each other. There are still ill feelings involving exes, and a ceremony involving family is a logistical and emotional nightmare waiting to happen. The very thought of it induces a wave of stress in my soul. Just because we two are giddy with excitement doesn't mean that a ceremony will be met with enthusiasm by others. The pressure would be intense. We conclude that it is best for all concerned that we have a simple civil service, just the two of us, to quietly become Mr. and Mrs. and go about our lives.

Looking at the calendar, we notice that a week from Tuesday will be Valentine's Day. Perhaps it's a little corny, but we immediately decide on the date. Jim jokes that at least he'll never forget our anniversary.

One other thing we're sure of at this point is who we want to perform the ceremony. As unlikely as it is, we want my boss, Larry, to do the honors. He's a licensed funeral director, but it just so happens that he's licensed to perform weddings, too. It makes for an unconventional wedding, we know, but we never did gravitate toward the expected.

The question of where remains open, but I figure I'd better ask and see if he is available on Valentine's Day first. We can worry about the location later. We're not really choosy about the details. At this point in our lives, it's all about the commitment we are making to each other, and we've already done that. It's the honeymoon that we need to work on – and fast. It's not easy to plan a nice honeymoon on such short notice, but Jim says he'll work on it first thing tomorrow.

For now we just want to enjoy the moment. Little about our lives will change, but we will be a married couple. I feel outrageously happy at the thought and as I putter in the kitchen, I chime in with Dean, "... *Ain't That a Kick in the Head?*"

The next morning at work I know I've got a bit of a smirk on my face, so I keep my head down. I don't want to spill my news until I have a chance to ask Larry if he'll officiate our wedding. His wife, Nancy, is sitting not too far away, so I know this is going to be exciting news for them. They've been cheering us on since we first met.

When he finally enters the room and visits me at my desk, I glance upward and try to wipe the dumb grin off my face. "Larry, will you marry me?" He does a double take and freezes momentarily, but Nancy gasps audibly.

"So you're really doing it?"

"Yes, would you happen to be free on Valentine's Day?"

He glances at Nancy and she smiles and nods her approval. "What time?"

"It really doesn't matter. We're open to suggestion."

And just like that, we've secured the date and officiant. Nancy asks where we plan to hold the ceremony. "We don't want a big deal. Just the two of us really, and we don't really know where to do it, maybe just at our house."

"How about our house?" Nancy is a natural-born hostess and party planner, and it shouldn't have surprised me in the least that she would make such an offer.

"But we really don't know too many people in town and we're not inviting anyone."

"Why don't you just leave it up to me? Even if it's a small service, it's your wedding and it should be special. We'll host it for you and make all the arrangements."

I am somewhat tentative about the whole thing and not sure how Jim will feel, so I tell her that I'll discuss it with him and let her know tomorrow. The important thing is, plans are progressing.

While that was going on, Jim was working on the honeymoon. He calls to ask if I would be interested in going to the Bahamas. Glorious sunshine, beautiful beaches ... what's not to like?

After work we exchange details. He agrees to let Nancy run with the ceremony however she sees fit, and I agree to the hotel and flight arrangements he worked up. With the push of a button, the honeymoon becomes a done deal.

"So, what are we going to wear?"

Jim's got a tux that he recently had tailored for his daughter's wedding, so I guess I've got to buy a new dress. The whole white bridal gown thing seems over-the-top, considering our decidedly non-traditional wedding plan. "How about red, for Valentines' Day?" Red it is then.

So now we're off to find wedding rings. As with everything else, this doesn't work out quite as expected. We love the tradition of matching wedding rings, but are not successful in finding a set that suits us both. I like understated, feminine jewelry, but none of the rings I like has a masculine version for Jim. He has rather large fingers that call for a ring of substance. The rings that look so great on his finger look completely ridiculous on mine. We don't have time for customization, so we decide to choose different styles altogether.

I pick a dainty-looking narrow gold band with small diamonds. It goes well with the emerald and diamond ring he gave me last year, and it's exactly what I had in mind. He chooses a wider, gold and platinum band with a black detail that compliments his hand perfectly. Another item is checked off the short "to do" list.

The dress is not easy, but there is no time for a special order or fitting. I finally end up in a bridal shop, where I purchase a red bridesmaid's dress off the rack, white high-heeled shoes, and a sheer white wrap. Now we're getting somewhere.

Nancy has been giving me little hints about our big evening, but keeping it mostly to herself. Since we're shunning tradition, no invitations go out, but a blanket invite is issued to all employees of the funeral home. Basically, we're just leaving it in her hands, hoping she doesn't go to too much trouble. There are plans for a video and photographs, and we picked a song to be played right after the "you may kiss the bride" part.

We told our kids first, then our parents and other relatives. It came as no surprise to anyone and our news was met with good wishes all around, blessings from the kids, and what we perceive to be a collective sigh of relief that they would not be expected to make arrangements to attend a formal ceremony.

There is little to do now but to think about what we need to bring to the Bahamas, ask the neighbors to tend to our cats in our absence, and anticipate the big moment.

No More Secs!

CHAPTER 11
"My Condolences … oops. You May Kiss the Bride"

It's our wedding day. The ceremony is scheduled for 6:00 p.m., and upon Nancy's insistence, I took the day off, even though I really don't need much prep time. I guess it just wouldn't seem fitting for a bride to spend the morning of her wedding in a funeral home.

I am stronger and healthier than either of us dared hope. The impractical white high heels I bought on a whim will not be an issue and I'm able to walk and move without the slightest difficulty. Standing through the vows will pose no hardship, and we are thrilled that I've managed to rebound so well. I don't need a cane and there isn't a single visible sign that I have MS.

We spend the day together at home with little fuss or fanfare. Without the stress and complications of a big wedding, we are able to concentrate on the matter at hand. Other than the fact that I'm having a bad hair day, everything is going along smoothly. I've long since given up on letting a bad hair day get in my way. That's something that definitely comes with age … or maybe I should say maturity.

We arranged to have a professional wedding portrait done before the ceremony, so we dress early and head to the photographer's studio. We really only want one good shot, but the photographer has us pose individually and together over and over again and suddenly I feel like a bride.

As we pull up to Larry and Nancy's beautiful home, we notice quite a few cars on the street. This can't possibly be for us. We don't know that many people in this town. The February air is chilly, and we are ushered in through the garage so we won't have to brave the February weather.

All smiles, Nancy immediately leads us off into an elegant bedroom, where she has arranged for us to spend a few quiet moments together before reappearing in the living room. Larry fills two champagne flutes that have been engraved with our initials and today's date, and they leave us to our private toast. We can hardly believe how generous they are being and how much they seem to be enjoying our happiness.

This is definitely more than we expected, and we are feeling very special, indeed. If you can't share happiness with family and old friends, then new friends and co-workers can fill the void. This is so good, so romantic and beautiful, that I can hardly believe this is real. We are living a mini fairy tale.

"Well, here's to you."

"To us." We lift our glasses in a toast. Jim looks superbly handsome in his tux and I feel lighter than air. My eyes are beginning to mist.

I believe I've made a triple play. Love. Intimacy. Friendship. I love him beyond all reason and feel loved in return. There is a powerful physical connection that cannot be denied. I genuinely like him as a person. If I weren't in love with him, I could definitely see us hanging out together. Forget triple play, this is a home run.

A quiet knock on the door and Nancy calls, "It's time!" This is our moment. We hold hands and emerge from the bedroom to a room filled with the funeral home staff and their spouses. I didn't expect so many of them to actually show up and I feel my first flutter of nervousness at the flash of a camera.

Flowers, candles, and assorted red valentine decorations fill the room and I'm stunned by the collective embrace I feel.

Larry welcomes us and the assorted guests and begins the ceremony. As he speaks I hear sniffles behind me, the clicking of cameras, and the whir of the video. This is really happening. My only fear is that I will be unable to recite my vows.

At Larry's prompting, Jim and I face each other and join hands. Jim, staring directly into my eyes, recites his vows first:

"I, James Marcel Pietrangelo, take you, Ann Linda, into my heart and into my life, as my wife.

Your grace, your beauty, your strength, your courage, your laugh, your capacity to love and to allow yourself to be loved, fuel the fire that burns in my soul for you.

I promise, in front of God and man, to be true to you in good times and in bad, in sickness and in health.

I will love you, protect you, and honor you for as long as I live, both in this life and in the next."

It's my turn and all my nervousness about memorizing the lines disappears as I lock in on Jim's serene face. I love this man and want to be his wife.

"Jim, you have seen me through some of the darkest and most painful days of my life with compassion, sacrifice and unwavering support.

You've been responsible for the happiest, most cherished moments of my life because of your charm, sense of humor, and the kindness of your heart.

I'm so proud and so honored to stand by your side today, to take your name, and to be united as husband and wife ... your partner in every way, through all the years of our lives.

I pledge to you companionship, passion, loyalty, respect, and love.

I give you my hand and I entrust you with my heart for as long as God allows us to be together."

"Wow," Larry whispers under his breath. More sniffles from over my left shoulder.

With the ceremony reaching its conclusion, Jim places his arm around my waist, pulls me in tightly, and delivers a long, soft kiss, solidifying the new union.

As planned, we indulge in a brief dance to "You Feel Good," a song by Tracy Byrd that begins by talking about sleeping in the nude. We laugh at our own ridiculous choice for a wedding song, but the words and the sentiment of the song fit the occasion perfectly.

If anyone present finds this whole thing a bit off, they are keeping it to themselves. Everyone is acting as though this a perfectly normal wedding.

"Mrs. P!" calls Nancy as she leads us into the other room, where she has arranged hors d'oeuvres and a beautiful little wedding cake, complete with an engraved cake knife.

The assembled group exchanges pleasantries and congratulates us. They can't possibly know how they have touched our hearts on this day. Perhaps we aren't so alone in Virginia after all.

I managed to get through the entire day without the intrusion or even the faintest thought of MS. Jim was so right to suggest that we strike while the iron is hot, so to speak.

Our wedding definitely falls in the category of "out there." No family was present, our rings didn't match, the bride wore red, and the officiant was a funeral director. Then again, quirky isn't necessarily a negative. The important thing is that our commitment to each other has been formalized.

It is at this point in fairy tales that we are generally told that the couple "lived happily ever after." But life isn't a fairy tale and marriage, we both know from previous experience, is anything but predictable. In the best case scenario, we've got a lot of years left on our journey together, a journey that could take us anyplace at all. There will be good, bad, and every conceivable variation in between. This time around, we are privy to the secret of it all – we will expect the unexpected and never, not for a single moment, take our union for granted.

Back home, we put the finishing touches on our packing. We cuddle up in bed, for the first time as husband and wife, and the world is a very different place. Mrs. P. It has a certain ring to it.

We took an early morning flight so we could be enjoying the ocean breezes of the Bahamas by midday. As we land I feel as though we are in a different universe altogether. The warm air, the sounds of the ocean, and the slower pace remove all distractions and encourage a laid back lifestyle.

When we reach our room, we are completely blown away. It is light and airy, with big windows and lots of room to stretch out. There's a box on our door and it is explained that in the morning we will find croissants and muffins for breakfast in there. What a charming tradition!

We waste no time in getting outside to walk the beach. I'm feeling so strong that I take off on a spontaneous little run, just because I can. It is one of those "look what I can do!" events. I laugh at my own childlike glee at such a simple thing as a short run on the beach. It's as if the universe set aside this time and this space just for us and I am deeply grateful.

We stroll the local shops at our leisure and enjoy the interesting architecture and colorful sites. We've got no particular schedule and are living for the moment.

The ocean is alive with life and so are we. Neither sunrise nor sunset ever looked as beautiful and I've never been more at peace.

One night we decide to take a sunset cruise. We arrive at a small boat just after dinner and are joined by several other couples. We take a slow cruise away from shore and stop to admire the sunset. It is a splendid display of gold, orange, and pink, and we all marvel at nature's beauty. We try to, but can't quite succeed, in capturing the moment on film.

The magic that we feel is about more than is painted in the sky. It's about the night air, the gentle wind, and the small talk with our fellow passengers. It's about the feeling of wholeness that we now possess. Nobody on this island would guess that I ever had a problem walking. But I do think they can guess that we are on our honeymoon. Ah, young ... er ... middle-age love.

Later, back in our room, we don the plush white robes provided by the hotel and snuggle up on the sofa. We leave the windows open to catch the evening breezes. We don't want to squander a single nanosecond of our honeymoon.

We haven't talked about MS since we've been here, but it is hardly something one can forget for long periods of time. We fully expect our lives to mirror the relapsing/remitting nature of MS. We'll alternate between husband and wife and caregiver and wife, and life will continue to challenge and amaze us. They say nothing is certain except change and we are living proof of that theory. Change is coming, so we are determined to take advantage of every opportunity to live to our full potential, whatever that potential may be at a given time.

Right now, we are soaking up the good life.

CHAPTER 12
Taking the Temperature

Dinner is quiet this evening, each of us lost in our private thoughts. I glance over at Jim and feel a rush of emotion as I clumsily twirl my spaghetti.

"Sweetheart, I want to talk to you about something."

Jim is finishing up his glass of Merlot and any minute now he's going to start clearing the table and heading for the sink. Not this time. Not if I can help it. Tonight I aim to head him off at the pass.

By all accounts, Jim's included, he has not always been so helpful around the house. It doesn't exactly fit in with the whole New Jersey Italian male thing. So what I'm about to do seems completely illogical, and is probably a symbolic blow to wives all around the world, but I've made up my mind.

"I know this is going to sound like an insanely ridiculous thing for a wife to say, but I would really appreciate it if you would stop doing the dinner dishes."

He looks slightly stunned, yet relieved that the matter was not a more serious one. Laughing, he asks, "Why wouldn't you want me to do the dishes?" Surely he thinks I've gone mad.

My eyes are starting to tear up. "Because you already do so much, and the dinner dishes are something I can handle, no matter how bad off I am. I've got the stool and I can take as long as I need. It's just that you move faster than me and always beat me to it. It makes me feel so guilty."

That old MS guilt is a force to be reckoned with. It's always ready to poke away at your self-esteem. It's not like I asked for MS, or that I enjoy my downtime, but I feel guilty anyway. I've got to be careful here. If there ARE things that I can do, then I can't allow myself to slack off. I figure that's a surefire way to fall into a trap and become increasingly dependent on my husband, something I desperately want to avoid. If I'm going to take more control, this is as good a place as any to begin.

Sometimes he must be my caregiver – we've got no choice about that. But if it is not absolutely necessary, then the caregiver must step aside and make way for the husband.

"Okay ... are you sure? Every night?" I most definitely detect a hint of glee in his tone. I picture the backflips he is performing inside his head.

"Yes, I'm sure. I can always manage the dishes – but if I can't, I'll ask you for help."

"Well, I'm not going to argue with you." He's smiling and giving me that look. We stand up to clear the table, and end up in an embrace. That's another tradition we've started. After dinner, there must be a hug and kiss before he exists the room. I love our little traditions.

"I've got to be the dopiest wife in the world. What kind of wife asks her husband to STOP doing dishes?"

"A wonderful wife."

I wipe my tears and suddenly feel uplifted. I did it! I don't care how stupid it might sound to other women. This is not a male/female, husband/wife thing. My husband is a gem and I'm not going to use MS to get out of a chore that I am perfectly capable of doing – not while there are so many I can no longer do.

I took control over one more thing, a thing that seems fairly insignificant but is, in fact, a big deal, the bonus being that I know that Jim hates doing dishes anyway. I am fighting dependence. I am saying, "I can do it." That's two chores I've vowed to complete every day – dinner and dishes. No matter what. Yes, it is good to have goals.

I let the sounds of classic rock seep into my brain as I wash the dishes and bask in my small victory over MS. *"Joy to the World ..."*

In the other room, Jim must be basking a bit himself. It's a double victory.

When the dishes are stacked and drying in the rack, I decide that I'd like to take a stroll around the neighborhood. Jim has a project to finish up, and it's been ages since I've walked the neighborhood alone, so I put on my walking shoes and tell him I'll be back shortly.

I'm walking wobbly right now, but I think I can leave the cane at home. I start down the driveway, which has an ever-so-slight incline, making me feel a bit unsteady. I keep my pace very slow in order to maintain balance and start off on my journey. I make it down our street and on to the next.

I can't really walk around a block, per se. Our neighborhood is a series of cul-de-sacs and dead end streets, so there is no block to speak of. We live in a pleasant area, with modest homes, lush greenery, kids on bikes, and barking dogs – a real slice of Americana. With no through roads, traffic is restricted to people who live nearby or their visitors.

As I tire, my gait changes and my legs get further apart, while my arms tend to flail about to the sides for balance. I don't want to make a spectacle of myself, so I decide to double back fairly quickly so that I can return to our driveway before my legs give me too much trouble.

Turning the final corner, my internal steering mechanism goes on the fritz and I start to lean left, until I'm actually in the middle of the road before I regain control. In retrospect, I should have brought my cane along. If there's anybody watching me, I'm going to look like a drunken fool if I abruptly turn right! I have no choice but to continue on my leftward trajectory and cross the road completely, as if that's what I intended all along. The trouble is, I needed to be on the other side.

The thought of it makes me start to laugh. Out loud. Oh, perfect. If anyone is watching, they will no doubt consider me a lunatic, but it's MS that ails me and at least I've managed to keep a sense of humor about the whole thing. There's probably nobody watching anyway, so I make the turn.

When I return home, I take my shoes off right away to calm the fire in my feet. I put my throbbing legs up on the sofa and let out a big sigh.

"How're you doin' babe?"

"I'm tired, but the walk felt good." It's been quite a day. All this introspection and soul searching can really tire a girl out.

The next morning I enter the kitchen and grab the medication that Jim left on the counter for me, choose a spot on my lower back, and self-inject. There's a little blood, and I use a square of cotton to tidy it up.

"I noticed you've been taking your shots without me these past few days. How come? Don't you want me to help you anymore?" Jim asked, looking slightly hurt.

"Well, I've been thinking about that a lot lately. I appreciate that you've been doing it for me all this time, but I need to take over. I don't want to get in the habit of you helping me too much, if it's something I can do myself."

As he usually does when I make such requests, he agrees to go along with me, although I think I see a hint of disappointment. I know he doesn't mind helping me out, but I really need to do as much as I can for myself for as long as I can.

I've given a great deal of thought to this strategy, and I'm finally taking steps to put it into action. I've never been much of a planner, living life by the seat of my pants for the most part. The very nature of MS hinders long-term planning, at least as far as details go, but general planning is something I need to keep in mind. Basic details must be considered, such as how I want to treat my symptoms medically, or whether or not I want to stay in my current job or aspire to something else.

The thing about relapsing/remitting MS is that your disabilities are ever-changing. You have to learn to adapt to new situations very quickly. Change is the name of the game. Finding a comfortable rut and staying there is just not going to happen. Reevaluation of life, taking the temperature, as Jim would say, is going to have to become the constant theme.

I'm warming up to the idea of change. In fact, I am at the point where I am ready for something major to change. For starters, I'm moving up to the driver's seat of my own life. Beyond that, I know there is something more that I should be doing, but I haven't quite got that figured out yet.

Ann Pietrangelo

CHAPTER 13
I've Never Seen That Before

I let out a long, low moan. From a sound sleep to intense pain in an instant. Now Jim is awake, too. "What's wrong?"

"My toe! It's one of those spasms again!" My whole leg, from my ankle to my knee is as tight as an overwound guitar string. "It's the big toe, and it's pointing up!" It is painful enough to bring a tear to my eye, but I'm giggling, too.

This is my third incidence with toe spasms. The first two times, we were just sitting around when the second toe of my right foot suddenly snapped into a complete downward position. It feels as though my whole foot is on the verge of spasming as well. Massage helps to bring it back into position, but it acts as if operated by an invisible spring. Walking is not possible.

Jim begins to massage my toe and foot, much to my relief. "Wow! I've never seen anything like this before. It's so tight, as if your toe wants to snap right off." I rub my calves while he works on the foot.

As soon as he pulls his hands away, the darn toe slams itself back into an upward position. "Ow! Ow!"

A few minutes of massage and I am released from the pain.

How strange it is, to have a part of your body do something without your permission. It's like being possessed by an otherworldly entity.

It's been a great three months, but I'm in the early stages of another relapse, this one involving new symptoms. I seem to have lost feeling in my mouth. Strange as it sounds, I've been biting the insides of my cheeks. I can't figure out how I manage to get my cheeks in between my teeth when chewing, but the bloody bite marks tell the tale. It's not very dignified, but at least it doesn't hurt.

It does hurt, however, when I manage to bite my tongue or lips. I've been chewing my whole life and all of a sudden, I can't manage the task without injuring myself. Eating salad is embarrassing, too. It slips down my lips, along with the oil and vinegar, and I find myself trying, without success, to scoop it all back in before Jim notices. I always prided myself on my good table manners and find this new state of affairs rather disturbing. Vanity requires that I not partake of salad for the time being. That and the desire to avoid choking.

I'm supposed to let the doctor know when I'm on the verge of another relapse, but this is getting ridiculous. When I finally got to speak to a human being on the phone and explained the reason for my call, I was told that I should eat an apple or something – I was probably feeling weak for lack of nutritious food like fruit. I was almost speechless, but not quite. I'm not suffering from low blood sugar here; I have multiple sclerosis. A piece of fruit? Really? Hey, everyone. The cure for MS is a piece fruit!

The return call was a suggestion for another round of steroids, but I hesitantly declined. Something about it just doesn't feel right and it is ridiculously expensive. And I definitely don't need the crazed state that made me tackle the great wallpaper project of last year.

I did agree to another MRI, also at the doctor's suggestion. He wants to see how I'm doing, as far as lesions are concerned. In a repeat of the last performance, Jim and I sit in his office as he calls in a colleague to review the scans with him. "I've never seen that before," he says.

"No, I haven't either." Uh-oh. Well that's not something anyone wants to hear in a neurologist's office, but something I've heard several times since, causing me to ponder whether I am actually of this earth or from outer space. I really must speak to my mother about that.

"Have you been exposed to metals?" he asks.

"Metals? No, not that I'm aware of."

"This looks like metal poisoning. Manganese, to be specific." You've got to be kidding me. I don't even know what manganese is. "But it could be just a bad MRI." The two doctors mumble to each other while trying to figure out exactly what it is they are looking at.

Here's where I engage in fantastical thinking again. Maybe I don't have MS. Maybe it's some kind of poisoning that they can flush from my system. Yeah, and maybe the tooth fairy is real, too.

Jim suggests that since they are not sure, perhaps we should just schedule another MRI, but they insist on testing me for a variety of metals, among other things. The doctor seems genuinely concerned and we are going to have to follow his hunch. I don't think manganese poisoning is something to ignore. I wouldn't be surprised if they suspect my husband is poisoning me.

I can't believe this turn of events, but now I have to endure another round of blood and urine tests, as well as another complete physical exam and more neurological tests. Let the games begin.

When we get home and do some research, we find that manganese poisoning is an occupational hazard for welders. I'm not a welder, never been a welder, don't know a welder. How is this even possible?

A week later, here I am at work, skulking the hallways with my bright red urine container, in which I am to collect 24 hours worth of urine. Well, isn't this a lovely new accessory? And I thought the red paisley cane was something! At least they match. I am completely and finally over my former need to fade into the background. I am often conspicuous now and getting used to it.

My arm is black and blue from the blood tests because, as usual, the nurses couldn't get into my tiny veins without collapsing them. I've missed more work and I'm close to full-blown relapse again.

MS is something I was just beginning to make my peace with, and now I've got to wonder about metal poisoning and God knows what else. I hate the doctor-go-round and I hate having to deal with insurers. Everything is so much more complicated than it needs to be and it all feels so impersonal and cold.

"Where would I get ... what's the word ... you know what I mean." Jim's pretty good at filling in the blanks, usually knowing exactly what I mean even if I can't find the words. It's happening on a regular basis now and it is very frustrating, to say the least. Research indicates that word recall is part of the long list of possible symptoms of MS. Great. On the other hand, maybe I'm just distracted, fatigued, or getting older.

It's not a terrible problem at this point, definitely something I can live with. I'm so worn out by the endless stream of tests and doctor visits that I decide to ignore this symptom for the time being. Pick your battles and all that. It's probably not the right thing to do, but I can't take on every single individual symptom and still manage to carry on a life. And it is living that I want to do, not symptom management.

All the test results finally make it in and there is no evidence of metal poisoning or any other underlying health condition aside from MS. Jim and I, while thrilled at the false alarm, are angry. The final verdict is that it was a lousy MRI, one that cost us thousands of dollars in out-of-pocket expenses and a month of needless worry. Why hadn't we insisted on a repeat of the MRI in the first place?

It will be months before all the bills and hassles with the insurance are complete and it was all such a waste.

We're tiring of the whole system of health management. No, we can't escape the MS, and no, we can't take total control over our health care situation. We must rely on doctors for their expertise and we must deal with the cubicle dwellers of the insurance company. We feel trapped in an endless cycle of "necessary" tests and the mindless red tape of the insurance company. Don't even get me started on the voice mail systems one must endure when calling not only the insurer, but the doctors, too.

"You have reached the office of Dr. So and So. Please press one for English, two for Spanish." One.

"Our hours are Monday through Wednesday from 10:00 a.m. until 6:00 p.m., and Thursday and Friday from 8:00 a.m. until 4:00 p.m. We are closed on Saturday and Sunday. If you are calling from a physician's office, press one. If you are calling from a pharmacist's office, press two. If you are a patient, press three." Three.

"If this is an emergency, hang up and dial 911. If you would like to schedule an appointment, or change an appointment, press one. Cancellations require a 24-hour notice. If you wish to fill a prescription, you must make an appointment. If you wish to speak to the nurse, press two. If you wish to speak to the billing department, press three." Three.

"Your call is important to us. Please remain on the line." Remaining on the line … remaining on the line … remaining on the line …

"The billing department is currently experiencing a high volume of calls. (There's a shock.) At the sound of the tone, please leave a brief message. Be sure to clearly state your name, date of birth, home address, phone number, insurance information, and reason for calling. Someone will return your call within 48 hours. Thank you for your patience."

When dealing with that sequence, you definitely do not want to press the wrong number because it leads to another series of options that don't apply and you can't get back. And forget hitting "0." They've got that booby trapped, too. And if they do call you back (maybe they will, maybe they won't), make sure you have all your paperwork handy because they will not have any of the information that you so clearly and patiently stated after the voice mail system prompt. The same kind of crummy system exists in the offices of the health insurers. It's enough to drive a person over the edge, and for me, that edge is getting dangerously close.

My insurance company has more control over my life than I do. That became crystal clear when I suffered a painful bout of frozen shoulder, something I'm told is in no way related to my MS.

After going through the required cycle of visiting a general physician first, then enduring some physical therapy even though the doctor didn't offer a diagnosis, and then waiting two months for an appointment with this orthopedic surgeon, he spent all of 90 seconds with me and left the room mumbling something about an MRI. "Oh, great," I thought, as I waited for him to return. "Another MRI. Why not just take my first born child now?" But he didn't return.

A nurse came into the room and announced, "You can go now."

"Isn't the doctor coming back?"

"No, you're all done!"

"But didn't the doctor say something about an MRI?"

"Oh, yes, but we have to contact your insurance company to see if you can have an MRI. If they approve, you will receive a letter by mail telling you when your appointment is." It was the bum's rush for me.

That's what we've come to. I'm just a shoulder that belongs to an insurance company. My input as to the next steps is not required. Do not ask questions. Do not pass go. Hell, I didn't even realize my time with the doctor was up. They could have saved us all a lot of trouble if the insurance company and the doctor just left me out of the equation all together. Maybe I could just drop off my shoulder at the drive-through next time.

I should point out that several years later, I would have the same problem with my other shoulder. I was fortunate enough to find a new orthopedic surgeon who treated me as a whole human being, kept the expenses to a minimum with a no-nonsense approach, and successfully treated the problem in short order. He was kind and did, in fact, put me in mind of Marcus Welby. Score one for the good guys.

We can't control the way the world works, but we can take back a certain amount of control over our lives. We can at least slow things down and make the process a better fit for ourselves. I'm not terminal – at least not more so than anybody else – and I'm not going to give myself over to constant monitoring and testing. From now on, I'm not going to take every test that is suggested unless there is good reason. I'm not going to take a new prescription for every symptom that comes along and with that, have new side effects to deal with. I will learn to LIVE with MS, not merely exist alongside it.

In our case, at least, the doctors we've dealt with have not had firm opinions on particular treatment options. They do love to schedule expensive tests, though. They inform us of possibilities and probabilities, but do not argue strongly in favor for or against anything, and I guess that is to their credit. MS is just too variable and unpredictable a disease. But since they are basically noncommittal, we're going to have to commit to something ourselves, and that something is going to be less intrusion, more living.

So we're starting with the steroids. We've lived through a couple of doses now, and were not at all pleased with the results, at least in the short term. Barring any new and horrifying symptoms – such as vision loss – I'm going to skip additional treatments. I'm going to hold off on any fatigue-fighting medications as well. The expense and the side effects do not balance out any gain at this time, but we'll keep all our options open should things change.

I recall the words of the nurse when I arrived at the hospital for my first round of Solu-Medrol, "You and I are going to be seeing a lot of each other from now on."

Until this point, I've been doing everything the doctors have told me to do. Try this medication, then try that one. Take this test, the results of which call for another test. Visit the general physician, the neurologist, the physical therapist, and specialists of every sort. It's not as though any of these things will make MS go away. What am I doing with my life? No, we're not going to be seeing a lot of each other. That is not the life I'm going to live.

I may have MS, but too much medical intervention is beginning to take a toll. I do not wish to become a perpetual patient. I just want to be a person who happens to have MS.

I'm certainly not going to abandon modern medicine. I will continue to see a doctor and for now will remain consistent with my use of the daily disease-modifying medication. Above and beyond that, there's going to be an entirely new approach. Life first, MS second.

CHAPTER 14
Untidy Chapters

We didn't plan on buying a wheelchair. I've only used them in airports and once borrowed the chair from the funeral home for an MS Society Walk. Jim and I had each been soliciting sponsors for two months, but as the day of the walk drew near, my latest bout with the beast was getting the best of me. There was no way I was going to cop out, but a wheelchair was our only choice. Jim would push me the entire length of the walk. I wasn't thrilled about it, but what better time to be seen in a wheelchair? So often the public face of MS is the healthy-looking sort, but the truth is that MS is not always so invisible.

Even as a last resort, I've got my problems with wheelchairs because when my legs go, so do my arms. It is not possible for me to propel myself, so someone must push me. If it ever comes down to me requiring one on a more permanent basis, it's going to have to be an electric model, but I am going to assume that will never be necessary.

On a routine Costco run, we spotted a lightweight, folding wheelchair. We'd spoken about the possibility of purchasing a wheelchair for "special" occasions, and we finally bit the bullet.

The lightweight chair in question will be perfect for travel or any future event that would require walking any distance. It doesn't have the larger wheels of most chairs, but four tiny wheels, and the leg braces are removable for easy stowage. It's a big step, buying this chair, but it is not the emotional torpedo it could be. After all, I don't need a wheelchair very often, and it is simply one more tool added to our arsenal to be called into duty as needed. For the most part, it will remain in a dark corner of our basement gathering dust, but fulfilling a purpose nonetheless.

More changes have come in small doses, some more obvious than others. No matter how you look at it, everything is different than it was before diagnosis, though not in an entirely negative way. Perhaps some of the changes that I casually attribute to MS are due to other circumstances. They may be changes that would have come even if MS had not entered the picture. It's no simple task to assign meaning to an individual event because, unlike the neat chapters in a book, or the absolutes of episodic television, life's ups and downs tumble around in no particular order or regard for what else is going on. New episodes begin even while old ones are in midstream and unresolved; some are forever unresolved.

Things don't happen in perfect, sensible succession. We can't take any situation and apply our understanding in a vacuum. Within the span of just a few years, in a rather untidy, overlapping manner, I ended a marriage and began a new one; for the second time in my life relocated to another state, leaving loved ones behind; hit my mid 40's; had to quit full-time work and phase myself into being a part-timer; got a couple of cats; and received a diagnosis of multiple sclerosis.

Also in that time period, we moved from one house to another in the same city; traveled around to visit family in other states; entertained house guests; celebrated graduations and weddings; worried, as parents do, about our offspring; and mourned the passing of loved ones. Oh, and I gained a few fine lines around my eyes. They give me character. Just because I have MS, doesn't mean that all other life events stop. They don't. Whatever the state of my health, life goes on around us and, ready or not, we've got to participate.

All that has resulted in a major shift in my attitude, my way of looking at the world, and the way the world looks at me – or at least my perception of how the world looks at me. I'm a much more patient person, more content, and more confident than I've ever been, even as I've lost some of the independence I so prized. To say that these changes are due to MS, or even to my new marriage, would be an oversimplification. There was just too much going on all at once to be able to pinpoint the hows and whys of it all. Of one thing I have no doubt – what I've gained is far greater than what I've lost.

With a fresh sense of introspection, I decide to express my feelings in writing. I'm comfortable on the keyboard, where I can pour out my deepest thoughts, things I find difficult to say aloud. I'd forgotten how much I enjoyed writing, how comfortable I am with the process. Given the choice, I've always preferred the written word to the oral conversation, where I can get tongue-tied and lose my train of thought. Maybe this is just the therapy I've needed.

Jim says I'm pretty good. He's such an amazing writer himself that his approval gives me a bit of a high. It seems that I've found a hobby, a pleasant pastime, one that Jim and I can share to a certain extent.

I still remember the first thrill I ever felt for writing. It was the early 80's and my mother was about to turn 50 years old. In honor of her birthday, I wrote something that I loosely refer to as a poem. Signed and framed, I presented it as her birthday gift. In true Mom fashion, she gushed appreciatively.

I showed the poem to some of my office pals and they liked it so much that several of them asked if they could use it for their own mothers. Flattered, I happily distributed my little work, going so far as to tweak the others to personalize them.

Looking back on it now, I don't think it was a particularly good poem, and I really haven't the vaguest clue how to write poetry. I don't even think it was a stellar piece of writing, but it had heart and made an impact. My words were powerful enough to touch not only my own mother, but others as well. That was the thrill of it all. I was in my early 20's then and loved playing with words and writing letters to friends and family, but certainly didn't see any future in it. To this day, that framed poem still occupies a space on Mom's bedroom dresser. Now I am beginning to understand that a writer has always dwelled inside of me – it's just taken a few decades to bubble up to the surface.

I recall that as a child I had romantic visions of being a writer. I longed to borrow my sister's portable Brother typewriter and be one of those interesting writer-types I'd seen in the movies, sitting in a lonely smoke-filled room with a pencil behind one ear and crumpled paper all over the floor.

Now I find myself returning to that familiar old fantasy and writing just for the sake of writing. I feel as though my life has been on hold these past few years while I waited for things to happen – and things have happened. But now it's time to MAKE things happen again. Maybe as I write the answers will come to me.

CHAPTER 15
Across the Pond and Out of Step

The plan was to sleep on the plane so that we would arrive fairly refreshed at 8:00 a.m. London time. The old saying about the best-laid plans is an old saying for a reason. Things aren't exactly going along as we hoped.

There is a screaming infant, but we should have anticipated that. There's always a screaming infant. What we really didn't anticipate was the level of discomfort in these coach seats.

Luckily, we've each had our own television screens with more than 50 movies to choose from, and were served decent meals. Neither of us has slept more than a few minutes and we are about to touch down. Every muscle in my body is aching and my feet are totally numb. My neck is so stiff I can barely turn, and it hurts badly. I refuse to complain; I'm not going to be that person. I'm in jolly old England with my handsome husband, for crying out loud, and I am going to make the most of every second.

As part of his duties as President of the AMOA, Jim and I are expected to attend a trade show, along with a few social functions. It's January, winter in the U.K., but it hasn't dampened our excitement. Jim has been here before, but this is my first trip to Europe and I'm more than a little excited.

We make it through customs rather quickly and grab one of London's famous black cabs that, although expensive, are particularly roomy and easy for me to maneuver. We can stretch to our hearts content, but I'm more interested in checking out my surroundings as we move through the crowded streets.

We make it to the hotel by 9:30 a.m. Unfortunately, it is too early to secure our room and we are both exhausted. We pull our luggage aside, grab a couple of chairs in the cavernous lobby, and settle in for the wait.

I can't take off my coat because it is freezing in here. The doors keep opening as guests arrive and depart, letting in more of the frigid morning air. Despite a crushing pain in my neck and difficulty staying awake, I'm enjoying some good old-fashioned people watching. It's one of my favorite past times.

When we are finally able to get a room, I am more than ready for a nap. We don't want to sleep too long, but a few hours of shut-eye will do us both some good.

After our nap, we shower and change. We've got nothing official planned for this afternoon and evening, and we decide to do a little exploring. I'm walking slowly these days and using a cane for balance, but I'm doing well enough to manage quite nicely.

We head outside to familiarize ourselves with the neighborhood and find nearby eateries. When the cold air hits my contact lenses, the waterworks begins. An eye doctor once told me that I have overactive tear ducts because my eyes are actually too dry. Unfortunately, the slightest breeze or ray of sunshine results in uncontrollable tearing. Whenever we're out in public, we wonder what people think about the crying lady with the cane.

It's not going to stop us from enjoying ourselves, though. One item at the top of my "to do" list is to sample the local fish and chips. I've got a thing for fish and chips.

Back in my hometown of Woonsocket, there is a hole-in-the-wall place called Ye Olde English Fish and Chips. It's the kind of place that, were you filming a movie about New England, would capture the feel and sense of place you would need to tell your story. It's not particularly impressive to look at, but show up on a Friday night and you may find yourself standing in a line outside, taking in the aroma and listening to your stomach growl. Patrons order at the counter for take out or dining in the casual booths. The air is saturated with the smell of fish and the diners are animated and speak in the southern New England accent that I never really heard until I moved away.

The fish is deep fried in plenty of batter and the fries are big and meaty. Throw in one of their giant dill pickles, and your taste buds never had it so good. After you've eaten the last fry with vinegar, you'll swear that you'll never eat again, but you know in your heart that you will be back.

Ever since I was a kid, I wondered if this flavorful delight really bore any resemblance to true English fare, and I will finally have my answer. Just two blocks from our hotel we spot it – a real honest to goodness English pub – with fish and chips on the menu. I can barely contain my excitement.

Upon entering the pub, we are immediately impressed with the decor of dark woods which give off a warm and friendly first impression. The place is packed with people who are obviously enjoying themselves.

If we're going to have fish and chips, I suppose we should have some dark English ale as well. I am not convinced that I will enjoy it, but I can't pass up the opportunity to try. The ale arrives first and I am stunned to find it chilled. I always heard the English take their beer warm. We are not big beer drinkers, but we find it refreshing and flavorful.

The fish arrives and it has the same thick, crispy-crunchy batter I know so well, although this fish still has the gray scales. It comes with fries, peas, and tartar sauce. It is love at first bite, and I will be able to report back to my Rhode Island family that their Ye Olde English is quite authentic, as far as I could tell. It is a delightful meal and I savor each bite. Imagine that ... I'm actually having fish and chips with ale in London!

Service is slower here; nobody seems in too much of a rush, and we soak in the atmosphere before heading back out into the cold to explore. London is a much more international city than I had imagined, a melting pot, really, with many foreign languages filling the air, and I feel my energy level rising with the hustle and bustle.

I was fascinated to find that there is a coffee shop on almost every corner. I always heard that the English don't care much for coffee, but of course, London is full of people from elsewhere, so it makes sense. There's no shortage of tea, either, and we have every intention of partaking in a relaxed afternoon tea while we are here. That charming tradition is something we will take home with us.

To my American eyes, the cars appear refreshingly tiny. Not an SUV in sight. They've got these cute little two-seaters that appear to have been cut in half right behind the front seats. I measured them to be the size of my arms held out straight to the sides, fingertip to fingertip, plus a couple of inches. I am unabashedly playing the American tourist and delighting in each new discovery. It's one thing to read about another place, quite another to experience it with your own senses.

The streets can be quite a hazard for foreign pedestrians like us. They drive on the left, but since I'm not driving, I didn't think that was something I had to worry about. Wrong! I didn't realize how that changes everything when you look both ways to cross the street. There are painted reminders right on the road telling us in no uncertain terms to "LOOK RIGHT" before crossing, but it's amazing how conditioned we are to crossing the street a certain way. A close brush with a passing vehicle serves as our wake-up call. Well, that ought to keep us on our toes.

The roadways are packed with cars, taxis, double-decker buses, bicycles, mopeds, motorcycles, and walkers. They all move together in an intricately choreographed dance, and I feel like Lucy in the chorus line – always a bit out of step.

We didn't spot any people with disabilities around, and hurried passersby paid little attention to my slow gait or my cane. Fellow walkers did not give way as they hurried toward their appointed destinations and I felt very vulnerable and out of place. Were it not for Jim spotting for me, I most assuredly would have ended up on the ground more than once. After some discussion, we decided that it would most likely be the same in any major city, and that we had just gotten used to a smaller town with more room to walk and more time for courtesy, not to mention more people with disabilities out and about. It was invigorating, yet a bit dizzying to be in the midst of it all.

Why is it that everywhere we go I am faced with stairs? In restaurants, the ladies' room always seems to be up a level, or down a level. Lucky for me that I have a strong bladder, because holding it is definitely easier than braving the stairs at this point. I just keep my liquid intake to minimum levels in these situations.

We braved the Tube at one point, but it was difficult to maneuver with confidence. Everything was moving way too fast for my comfort.

The next few days are a whirlwind of activities – the trade show, a tour of Westminster Abbey, Big Ben, Harrods Department Store, The Drury Lane Theatre to see *The Producers*, the changing of the guards at Buckingham Palace, afternoon tea, bangers and mash, more fish and chips, and the very formal trade show ball, where I was delighted to show off my lovely form-fitting gown chosen especially for this occasion.

At events where dancing is involved, I generally opt for "chair dancing," unless it is a slow dance where Jim can hold on to me and keep me close. I have two forms of chair dancing. When I am really struggling, I remain seated, but move my upper body and arms with the beat. If I'm a bit stronger, I stand behind the chair and hold the back while dancing. It helps me to feel like part of the action. All in all, well worth the effort.

Tonight we are scheduled to attend a cocktail party at a small art museum. I am beside myself with excitement as I slip my little black dress over my head and shoulders. It feels a little tight as Jim moves in to zip me up. Excitement quickly turns to panic as he lets loose with a soft whistle and I realize that the dress, when zipped, barely makes it over my backside! Oh, why hadn't I tried it on before packing? Just a few months ago, it looked so darling on me. Amazing what two or three pounds can do. All right, maybe five. I've got my size six butt in a size four dress and I sense disaster looming.

So now here I stand in my stupidly high heels, leaning on my cane, and wearing a dress that is straining at the seams. Out of time and options, we head out into the winter chill to hail a cab. As if having MS and walking with a cane in high heels weren't challenging enough, the tight dress is exaggerating my awkward gait to the point of ridiculousness. I'm the president's wife, for crying out loud. What kind of impression will I make?

After removing my coat at the museum, I carefully situate myself with my back to the wall, doing everything in my power to avoid mingling. When a chair becomes available, I sit down warily, hoping I won't split my dress open in the process. "It's all good," I think, nothing at all unusual about a person with a cane taking a seat. No reason for anyone to question it. Stay confident, now.

After cocktails, it is announced that the unveiling of a particular piece of art will take place on the second floor, and would all attendees please follow the guide upstairs. Stairs? We inquire as to the location of an elevator. No elevator? Well, isn't this a fine mess.

With my MS acting up, there is no way I can possibly make it up that long, wooden staircase in this ill-fitting dress without attracting curious eyes straight to my behind. Jim returns from a bit of mingling and I inform him that I am going to remain glued to this chair regardless of what he or anybody else does or says. Up to this point, he has been good-naturedly playing along with me, and now he is barely containing his laughter.

The moment the last of the partygoers makes it to the top of the stairs, we both start to laugh at my predicament. Courteous museum staff, spotting the cane, inquire about my difficulty with the stairs. "Multiple sclerosis," we tell them, with all the seriousness we can muster. Tears are falling from my eyes now, due to suppressed laughter, but no doubt mistaken for despair. Drinks and hors d'oeuvres are delivered with sympathetic smiles directly to our lonely corner.

Embarrassed and unable to control my laughing/crying, we skulk out the door at the very first opportunity. For once, MS actually rescued me from a "tight spot."

It's the morning of our departure from London, and my legs are not doing well. There is some kind of a computer glitch, causing the security line to be several hundred people strong.

Jim found me a seat and stood in line at the airline counter to explain my problem. Before long, we are provided with a wheelchair and an escort who will take us through security in short order. Unfortunately, our gate is still a long way off. A passing airport cart stops to offer me a lift and we gladly accept. But rules are rules, and they won't allow Jim to ride with me even though there is ample room. So off I go in the cart while Jim makes the long trek on foot to our faraway gate. I watch him trail behind, trudging through the airport crowds while I ride. As relieved as I am to rest, I feel that the caregiver is like Rodney Dangerfield – no respect. Regardless, Jim does not seem terribly ruffled.

At last, we are settled in on the plane and waiting for take off. It's been a whirlwind week and we're both exhausted. We've shared some wonderful quiet times together, some quite comical moments and, not incidentally, represented the trade association overseas – with a certain flair.

I am truly amazed by the quiet way my husband goes about the business of protecting me and trying to make life with MS more tolerable. This trip was proof positive that it pays to think things through as much as possible beforehand, but to be flexible and spontaneous in dealing with the daily changes that come with MS. With some planning and flexibility, we are able to work around obstacles that arise. It's okay to be slightly out of step. Of course, a good sense of humor helps.

CHAPTER 16
Hitchcock Could Have Written This

I let out a bloodcurdling scream as I bolt straight up from a dead sleep. The room is spinning wildly and the bed is lurching side to side, threatening to dump me off the side. I clutch at the bedding, trying to hold on, aware that I am on the verge of vomiting.

The house is dark, but I am conscious of Jim's presence beside me, trying to steady me and assess the situation. Instinctively, I realize that the room is not really spinning, nor am I possessed by demons, but for some reason, my body is convinced otherwise. I'm moaning and just short of panic, and Jim likely is, too. He turns on the lights and holds me upright.

I try to explain that I understand that nothing is really moving, but the spinning is making me sick anyway. "Maybe I should take you to the emergency room."

Oh, please, not that. "Let's wait. It's starting to calm down a bit. What time is it, anyway?"

"3:00 a.m."

I sit up, as still as I can, until I convince Jim that I'm okay. Fifteen minutes later, the movement has subsided. "I don't know what that was all about, but I think I'm better now. I'm sure it's nothing." I try not to let on how scared I am and assume he is doing likewise.

Finally, we turn off the lights and try to get back to sleep. Within minutes, the wild spinning resumes and I sit up again, trying to quell the nausea. Every fiber of my being tells me that the room is spinning and moving up and down, but intellectually, I understand that it is not so. How can this be? Jim is beside himself with worry. The pattern repeats itself over and over until the first light of morning. What is happening to me now?

At 9:00 a.m. sharp, Jim is on the phone with the doctor, who has no difficulty pinpointing this new craziness as a classic case of vertigo. He says not to worry, but to try an over-the-counter medication. So *that's* vertigo!

It's 11:00 before I feel back in control of my physical senses, and I've missed another morning of work. As has been my habit, a new symptom sends me on a mission to research and learn. The first thing I learn about vertigo is that it has nothing to do with fear of heights.

My only reference to vertigo until now was Detective Ferguson, excellently portrayed by Jimmy Stewart in Hitchcock's classic 1958 thriller, *Vertigo*. The film played on Ferguson's fear of heights, zeroing in on him as he reaches the third step of a ladder and is overcome with dizziness and collapses in a near faint. Hitchcock used unique camera angles and imagery to capture the fear of heights as never before. Excellent film, but not a good reference for true vertigo.

Vertigo is the sensation of extreme movement when there is none, and is a very common symptom of multiple sclerosis. The fact that it first hit during deep sleep turns out to be common as well. The only real danger is injury due to fall.

We learn that vertigo can be combated by turning the lights on, so that the eyes can signal the brain about your true surroundings, and by sitting with your back straight and head forward, with little movement. Getting comfortable in a recliner rather than the bed is a huge help.

At my next doctor visit, we are told of several prescription medications to combat vertigo, but we take a pass. It's something that comes and goes, and I plan on using the techniques I've learned that don't involve more medications. Now that we understand what is happening, it is infinitely less frightening. Most of the time, it passes very quickly.

Another symptom, another adjustment. Constant change means constant readjustment. As new symptoms appear, some old ones lay dormant. I haven't bitten the inside of my cheeks in months. I've reached the point where I can simply face each day with its unique challenges to the best of my ability. Certainly, there are a lot of people who have it worse than me. In the great scheme of things, I am really quite fortunate.

A few days later, Jim was not so fortunate. I returned from work to find him flat on his back on the floor of our office, clearly in agonizing pain. "My back went out – it's bad. I can't move."

It is startling to see him in this vulnerable state. Jim is a strong man, not just in spirit, but physically. His solid, muscular physique gives him the appearance of one who needn't be concerned about such things.

Once a year or so his back gives out and he's out of commission for awhile. It's as crippling and painful as anything I've ever seen and I never know quite how to help.

When the day comes that his back and my MS decide to get together, it's not going to be pretty.

Fortunately, I am in a good place right now, able to work, walk without a cane, and drive. It's a good thing, too, because I've got to drive to the drug store to get his prescription.

It's strange, this role reversal. Here I am in the pharmacy, waiting for his medication, and worrying about him at home all alone. I feel like an impostor in this role. I see a person with any kind of disability and I think, "You don't know it, but I'm one of you." Anyone looking at me today would see no trace of illness or disability. Sometimes I feel as though I don't know myself at all, as if two separate individuals reside within my brain, and perhaps they do.

I imagine Jim at home, still on the floor, kicking himself for being in the position of needing my help. Things look startlingly different from this angle. It's natural, when you are the patient, to wish you were the strong one. The flip side is that it's a horrible thing to have to watch someone you love suffer, knowing there is little you can do to help. Even though such moments are short-lived in our home, it is enough to teach me that Jim's job as my husband/caregiver is no easy task.

You'd think I'd feel better on this side of things, what with being able to get around and do things for him for a change. But it hits hard that no matter what I do for him, I cannot lessen his physical pain and discomfort; I can't do anything about the stress he feels regarding falling behind on his work, or having his wife tend to him. He's always the rock, the protector, and he takes that responsibility very seriously.

That's a role I simply cannot fill. I can do things for him, I can take care of some of his immediate needs, but I cannot offer the same level of security that he offers me in similar circumstances. I am not physically strong enough to even help him up off the floor should the need arise. Even as he does his best to avoid moving and aggravating his back, he is always conscious of the fact that a lot of responsibility rests exclusively on his shoulders.

A few nights later, as we sit in the living room to watch television, he squirms to get into a more comfortable position, clearly frustrated with the slow process of healing.

"It's a terrible thing when your body won't do what it's supposed to do!"

Both his voice and his expression confirm his agitation. It appears that he is actually on the verge of anger. The irony of his statement is not lost on either of us and a moment later, he flashes a slightly guilty smirk and says, "Yeah, I know, I know. I'm just so aggravated."

"I get it, hon." And I do. You live for 40-plus years with some sense of what your physical self can and cannot do and suddenly your body is a cantankerous stranger, turning on you. You tell it to do something and it refuses to obey. It moans and groans as if you are asking for the world and makes its displeasure known with no room for doubt. It's easy to take a body for granted when we are young and healthy. It's shocking when that same body, like a rebellious teenager, no longer allows you to boss it around. It is an all out mutiny.

It's not that Jim is a bad patient. In fact, he asks for little and makes it clear that he doesn't enjoy hovering. He'll tell me if and when he needs something. But from where I'm sitting now, this is much harder to take than when I am the one who is out of commission. If this is how it feels to walk in Jim's shoes, I have a newfound understanding of life from his perspective, and an even stronger respect for him.

Unplanned as it is, it is the perfect time for me to ponder our situation and look toward the future. I've been working hard at maintaining some sense of independence, challenging myself to push to my fullest potential each and every day. I know now that I can do more, *be* more.

Sometimes the pent up frustration from lack of direction puts me in mind of another Hitchcock thriller, *Psycho*. Not the stabbing part ... the anxious music part.

I can't take a nine to five job. That would surely be more than I could handle on a daily basis, and would lead to disaster when they realize how often I need to call in sick.

On the other hand, it doesn't mean that there is anything wrong with the job I have. It's only half a day and requires little physical effort. I'm comfortable there, and they are comfortable with my situation. No need to rock that boat.

That leaves me with another option. Maybe there is something I can do from home, something that would spark my imagination a bit and give me the feeling of accomplishment I've been searching for. It's the obvious choice.

My MS, while certainly an intrusion in our lives, has not led to major disability. I am not ready to give up on work and call it a day, even though some people have suggested that I should. I'm just not there yet, and I don't see any need to rush things.

I had more than 40 years of relatively good health. That's substantially more than a lot of people get, and I am very grateful for those years. So they ended faster than I would have hoped, but I am hardly in a position to complain about it. I often think about people who are paralyzed, and the emotional and physical toll on them. I relate because when my MS is at its worst, movement is very difficult, but it passes eventually.

Whether from progressive MS, some other condition, or spinal cord injury, they are in that wheelchair for life, without hope of walking away. That takes a certain emotional adjustment that I, at this point, have trouble wrapping my head around, because I get to keep climbing back out. My adjustments would be a welcome trade to a great many people. Thinking about that makes me realize how truly fortunate I am and how much I have going for me.

I'm not as healthy as I once was, but I'm doing well. I have a husband who loves and respects me, and children and stepchildren who are doing very well for themselves. I have a home – not just a house, but a home. Life is good, even with MS dive-bombing us at every opportunity.

I want to focus on learning to live a productive life with MS, and possibly even using this major life change to better myself and to do some good in the world. Exactly how to do that still eludes me, but thinking about it is becoming a full-time job. Even though I can't put my finger on it yet, I am confident that I'm going to find the answers I seek.

Ann Pietrangelo

CHAPTER 17
Shape Changing Ninja

"Let's go out for Chinese food tonight."

Yes, it has been awhile since we visited our favorite local Chinese restaurant and we are due to put in an appearance. How it became our favorite is still a mystery to us. I get the feeling that we didn't choose it, but it chose us.

We began dining there a few years ago and never intended to make it a regular thing. The owners/servers don't speak English well and come off as rather abrupt; the booths are uneven and uncomfortable; and they don't seem to understand the difference between fast take-out food and more leisurely dining.

We often find ourselves laughing at the unintentionally outrageously efficient service. Before we even take a seat they are on top of us, "You know what you want?" Before we can crack a menu, the order pad is out.

The food is served quickly and the plates are piled impossibly high with food that is over-the-top hot. For a die-hard Seinfeldian like me, this place is "The Chinese Restaurant" meets "Soup Nazi." It makes me kind of wish I was a comedy skit writer.

Something keeps calling us back to this place, and we've been regulars for years. It took some time, but we are familiar faces now, greeted with friendly hellos and smiles. In a weird way, this place has become our place, and we wouldn't have it any other way.

After a typical dinner there, I leave with a doggie bag. The huge delicious meals are entirely too much for me, so I always come away with tomorrow's lunch. With the prices they charge, it's quite a bargain.

Even though we've just eaten and consumed a pot of tea, I want to snuggle into some pajamas. I am exhausted to my very core.

The kind of fatigue that comes with a chronic illness is hard to describe if you've never experienced it. It's not about being sleepy or sluggish. It's not the kind of fatigue you feel if you've missed out on one good night's sleep or had a particularly harrowing day. It's not the afternoon slump that can be relieved by a cup of java.

It's an all-over heaviness that makes it difficult to move; it's a fogginess that drapes itself over you and prevents you from functioning normally; it's a complete and total inability to fight sleep. It is debilitating and often the most troubling symptom of MS. It is turning out to be my biggest foe.

This level of fatigue will occupy your mind with a strange train of thought. Just how much energy will it take to walk over there to pour yourself a glass of water? Or to call a friend, or to engage in conversation? Even laughing takes energy, this much I know for a fact. Don't let my face fool you. I'm laughing on the inside.

You've only got so much energy before your reserves are depleted. The trick is to try to gauge the levels and pace yourself. It is no easy task. It's like having a car with a broken fuel level gauge.

Even a visit from the kids can't vanquish this foe. I fall asleep sitting up, I nod off during conversation, I have trouble focusing my attention. Mind over matter is not going to win this particular battle.

If I could choose one single MS symptom and one alone to be rid of, it would be this mind-numbing fatigue that plagues me of late. Besides having to function in this world with that type of fatigue, a genuine frustration stems from not being understood. It is one of the invisible symptoms of chronic illness that makes other people question you and, on occasion, causes you to question yourself.

The fatigue is visible on my face, but usually misread as sadness, anger, or lack of interest. That troubles me. When my MS fatigue hits, I show up at the funeral home, take my seat, and get to work with little fanfare. There isn't an ounce of energy to spare, so I concentrate on the task at hand. Even office banter is sometimes too much effort and I hate to think that I come off as unfriendly or unsociable, but I'm pretty sure I do. So be it. It's another of those "appearances can be deceiving" things.

The literature on MS will give you tons of information about the physical symptoms of the condition, but nothing can adequately prepare you for the emotional toll of this on-again, off-again shape changing ninja called MS.

When the fatigue ends, people generally notice the change. They find me to be happier, more bubbly, more approachable. But I have no great news to share, nothing exciting going on here. And nothing about me has changed except that the fatigue and the fog that goes with it have lifted for the time being. There's nothing new about me at all, it's just me minus the fatigue. The real me, the old me, the non-MS me. Actually, I'm not at all sure which me is the "real" me anymore.

Coming back from the fatigue is not without its own set of problems. There is so much to catch up on, both physically and emotionally. The trouble lies in not knowing. Not knowing how long you've got before the ninja returns ... or how best to manage your time ... or in how to readjust to a normal routine, whatever that is ... or how to avoid overdoing in your newfound exuberance. MS has definitely tested and improved my time management skills.

I'm back, at least for awhile, but the fatigue seems to have a cycle of its own, unrelated to my other symptoms and relapses. It is very frustrating to have the arms and legs finally working only to crash with fatigue.

The almost perfect cyclical nature of my relapses and symptoms is slowly unraveling. It is all much less predictable and some symptoms remain during periods of remission. I seem to have mini relapses in between the larger ones. My overall strength and stamina are waning, but if change is a constant, then I will assume that things can change for the better again at some point.

We decided to invest in a laptop, and I am amazed at how much I love this thing! Sometimes I have trouble maintaining comfortable positioning at the desk and this little beauty means that I can lounge on the sofa, on our little deck, at the kitchen table, or even in bed. I can put my legs up and relax and still play around on the web or with my writing.

Fatigue or not, this small purchase, along with wireless Internet service, has the power to keep me connected, entertained, and involved. I'm becoming a bit of a shape changer myself.

CHAPTER 18
A Fairy Tale in the Midst of Chaos

Settling into the Tennessee Williams suite at the spectacular Monteleone Hotel in New Orleans, our conversation is about the city and the overall state of the area. It's been six months since Hurricane Katrina and broken levies devastated much of the gulf region. As president of AMOA, Jim chose to hold his mid-year board of directors meeting in this city. Having spent six years living and working in the area, he has a real love for the city and its people and felt strongly that groups like AMOA need to do more than just raise money, which they did to the tune of over $100,000. They also need to support the local tourism industry that is so important to the area. Despite a number of objections, Jim decided to put his faith in the local people and take them at their word that they would be able to pull it together enough to make it happen.

We rented a car and decided to drive around to see how the area has fared since Jim's last site inspection. Some areas showed no evidence of the storm, other streets showed varying levels of damage. It's disconcerting to drive down the road and to have a ten-foot-high water line running alongside you, marking signs, buildings, telephone poles, and pretty much everything else along the way.

Over the last several months, some trash and debris has been cleaned up, but mountains of stolen memories remain piled high in the wide medians separating roadways. Refrigerators, 10-20-30 or more, line the streets waiting to be collected, a sad reminder of what was lost. Most of the streets are now clear, but, with crater size potholes and manholes having erupted out of their former confines, it's hazardous driving if you're not paying attention.

Homes, at least what remain of many, stand as testament to the powers of wind and water. Every so often, we spot small clean-up crews, men and women cutting, bagging, hauling debris from here to someplace else. We marvel at their ability to work and not appear disheartened. Tackling tasks that, when measured against what is a much larger backdrop of destruction, must test even the most fervent believers. Truthfully, I expected to see more FEMA trailers. I'd heard so much about them on the news. But there were nowhere near as many to be found as I originally supposed. Red tape, I was told. The trailers are stacked up in staging yards, but it's not quite so easy to get one as you might imagine. A disjointed jumble of feelings, political, sociological, stirs in our bellies while we try to make sense of what we're seeing.

The Tennessee Williams suite at the Monteleone Hotel. As wonderful as that sounds, there is a certain amount of guilt to living this well while in the midst of chaos. The Monteleone's world-famous Carousel Bar is a fun gathering place for the AMOA group. Like a real carousel, the bar s-l-o-w-l-y circles the room and even the bartenders, who remain on a stationary platform. Believe me, if you already have balance issues, sipping a margarita or two at the Carousel Bar can be a really weird experience.

The following morning, after a brief breakfast meeting, Jim and I head out to tour the ninth ward, where we witness indescribable destruction and despair. Fats Domino had a house there, but it now stands ruined.

We then proceed on to Chalmette, a sleepy town just east of New Orleans where one of the board members lives. He took a small group into his parents' home, which, during the flood, was completely underwater. I stayed in the van, not wanting to expose myself to the mold and Lord knows whatever else still survived in there. Jim insisted that I wait behind, anyway, then went in himself. He is friends with the folks who own the home and wanted to get a sense of what happened. He emerged somewhat depressed.

Chalmette. It might as well have been called the end of the world. Because that's what it looked like. We navigated the streets carefully, the van slowly maneuvering around trees and cars that still littered the road. In one surrealistic moment, we had to actually turn around and go back the way we came. There was a completely intact house sitting smack in the middle of the road. It had literally been picked up and moved down the street by the power of the flood when the levies broke.

Trees everywhere – dead, gray, and lifeless, but still rooted and standing as eerie remnants of a past life. Street signs are missing. Traffic signals don't work. Electric and phone wires droop uselessly.

Cars, some abandoned, others looted and destroyed, can be found in the oddest places. Boats appear out of nowhere. Every so often, a car parked near a FEMA trailer or partially standing home can be found with spray paint pleadings of "do not tow or move this vehicle – not trash!" That really got to me.

Each time you pass what was once someone's home, broken, destroyed, the faded markings of tired rescue workers on the front door testifying to whether or not the house was searched, or bodies found, you find yourself reflecting on the fragility of your own comfortable existence. There but for the Grace of God ...

From this vantage point, any problems we have seem rather small. As the week wore on and we were in a position to speak to the people who witnessed Katrina's wrath, the human tragedy became less of an item on the news and more of a reality. Most of the French Quarter was unscathed, and we were able to enjoy such local delights as Cafe du Monde, Tujaques, the Pelican Club, Giovanni's, Arnaud's, lunches in sequestered courtyards, and the Quarter's unique art galleries, although they were considerably less crowded than days of old. A few hearty street performers did their best to entertain and make a living.

The next day some of the ladies and I decide to kill a few hours in a shopping mall. About 30 minutes into the trip I take advantage of a bench to rest my weary legs while my companions continue on with their shopping.

A slow-walking elderly man of slight build finds his way over to the bench, but he doesn't take a seat. Instead, he remains standing in front of me and begins to speak. I am terrible with foreign languages. Other than the fact that he is speaking an oriental language, I am clueless, and try to convey that.

He's talking numbers now. Something about a thousand, I think, or maybe a hundred, but I'm still not getting the picture. He keeps gesturing toward me with his index finger and talking about numbers. He doesn't seem to care that I don't understand him.

Finally, he leans over and, now much too close, rubs his hand gently along my arm. I am totally creeped out now, as it is finally sinking in that this little old man is offering me money to ... well, make his afternoon a little more pleasant.

Out of nowhere, one of my shopping buddies ambles up and lets out a "hey!" That's enough to send the old lecher on his way and turn my face crimson. I am momentarily frozen at the thought of my slow assessment of the situation before we start laughing at the ridiculousness of it all.

I've never been taken for a hooker in my life, and I am shocked to be taken for one now. Let's face it. A 40-something-year-old woman with a cane who is wearing modest capri pants and conservative blouse doesn't exactly fit the stereotype. What was this guy thinking? Or maybe I'm devastatingly captivating beyond all reason.

Who knows? Maybe that particular bench in that particular shopping mall is a "special" meeting place. Maybe I unwittingly occupied the hooker zone and maybe the guy thought the cane was part of a sex game. And maybe, despite my age, I'm still a bit naive. In any case, it's just plain freakish.

One day, lunch with the ladies took an interesting turn. We had just taken the first bites of our meal when we heard a noise from above. Looking up in unison, we saw the ceiling beginning to let go right over our heads. Four of us were able to move out of our chairs fairly quickly, one lady jumping right over the wrought iron gate behind her. The fifth woman was wedged in and literally froze in place as a ceiling fan let go and began to fall, along with a few ceiling tiles, making quite a commotion.

When we looked up again we saw that the ceiling fan, connected to a large metal box held up by wires, was dangling right where we were sitting and stopped only a few feet from the ground – right about head level when seated.

When the immediate danger passed, we glanced around the room to find that this incident was restricted to our table area only. The rest of the diners remained seated – but staring at our little group. Thankfully, no one was hurt.

Living up to its motto, "the city that care forgot," the New Orleans eatery continued to serve without missing a single beat. If Katrina didn't stop them, a little ceiling fan incident most definitely would not. We politely declined another table and thanked the waiter for comping our meal. Instead, we took a few photos and headed back to the Carousel Bar to tell the guys of our adventure.

By the end of our trip, meeting attendees were thanking Jim for sticking with New Orleans, feeling richer for the experience. I concur. These wonderful people, feeling forgotten by the rest of the country, deeply touched my heart and made me grateful for my many blessings.

What I felt there is something that would stick with me always, further proof that uncertainty is part of living. Other than this very moment, what do we know? None of us has a crystal ball into the future and change comes when it comes, ready or not. Lack of a road map is most assuredly not unique to my life. Human beings just do not come equipped with a GPS.

CHAPTER 19
Crossroads

I look over at Jim as he sleeps. He is face down, arms underneath his pillow. The curve of his shoulders and the sound of his breathing fill me with a sense of contentment that is hard to describe. I stare at him for a long time before turning away and curling my body into his.

He stirs and I feel his body move. With one arm, he gently pulls me closer into a spoon position. He often holds me this way in the morning, giving me the feeling of being surrounded by his love. It is a cocoon-like state that allows me to fantasize that the world no longer exists and that nothing or no one could ever intrude. I am grateful for the simple pleasure of loving and being loved.

Being the husband of someone with MS is obviously no joyride, but I've never heard a complaint. Most of the time, I'm able to take care of myself and my responsibilities, but when I'm not, that's when Jim kicks into high gear.

Sometimes, "Hey, babe ... how're you doing out there?" simply doesn't cover it. Just as the pebble thrown into the pond begins a ripple effect, so does MS in the family. It reaches out in an ever-widening circle until it touches every aspect of your lives.

Jim's tenure as president of the AMOA is winding down, and we've known for quite some time that his association with IDS would not last, but that didn't make it any easier when the time finally arrived. With a lifetime of experience in sales, marketing, distribution, and running various start-up businesses, Jim finds himself in an uncomfortable position. He has to consider what his next move will be, career-wise. That can be difficult in and of itself, but now I'm part of the equation ... me and MS.

He's seen me through the worst of my relapses and knows exactly how bad things get. He also knows that without family in the area, I rely on him completely. Now, as he ponders his next move, he's got to keep that in mind. A highly demanding job or a position that requires extensive travel could prove to be too much for us. Who will look after me when he's busy or on the road? And what of my job? Without him to drive me when I can't drive myself, that's another thing that will have to go.

We were going to be the Dream Team. That was the plan, anyway, together in all things. Choosing the wrong career path would mean that the dream is at risk. We're going to have to make some very difficult choices, but we know that the core of our lifestyle must not be tampered with.

A lot can happen with MS in a few years. Neither of us is getting any younger and we are determined to enjoy our lives together to the fullest while the MS is still a manageable monster.

Like many men, or so it seems, Jim has always been fascinated with the latest technology. No matter how busy he was with goings-on at work or home, he always dabbled with computers and somehow managed to acquire all the latest gadgets. In college he took a computer course, back in the days when that meant programming on punch cards and when the 'computer room' was a huge, sealed environment and you needed to make an appointment to use one of the terminals. He completed that semester course in less than six weeks and still remembers his professor trying to talk him, unsuccessfully, into switching his major from business administration to computer science.

Following a period of deep introspection and careful consideration, Jim decided to change gears and try to make a living working with computers.

Several years ago, Jim formed a company, WebCamp One, LLC, but, until now, had really not made much use of it. With the economy starting to falter and the coin-op industry losing ground to an avalanche of home-based recreation products, he decided to dive head first into the world of freelance web development. It was a bold – some would say foolish move – full of risk. But for us it made a lot of sense. This would allow Jim to work from home and not have to travel as much as he did in the past. My MS is unpredictable in the frequency, duration, and severity of attacks, and, with no family nearby to count on during those times, Jim wanted to make sure that whatever he decided to do about work, he would be there for me when I need him.

Now all he had to do was improve his skills to the point where he could move from amateur to professional status. Somewhat amazing to me is Jim's ability to read books and teach himself new things. And that's what he did. Between taking some online classes and devouring a library's worth of books about web design, Jim built up the confidence to advertise his services. With each new project he gained experience and confidence, but it wasn't until he was asked to solve a rather tricky layout problem for the folks building a website for the Pulitzer Prize that he had an understanding of just how good he had become.

Nonetheless, the decision to enter the world of web design and development was a decision not without consequences. We will continue to question the saneness of that decision for years to come.

We're also discussing moving. Without IDS, we really have no ties to the area. With our children and families scattered about as they are, we are hard pressed to decide where "home" is, but we realize that we need closer family ties and a sense of community.

My COBRA coverage will be ending soon and that is another problem added to the mix. Health insurance regulations are a tangled mess, different for every state, and I've got a whopping pre-existing condition. It is a huge consideration when you want to make a move but have no group insurance waiting for you on the other end. We're still only seeing the tip of this iceberg.

It's all up for grabs. With multiple loose ends, our daily conversation is peppered with musings about where to live and how best to approach career moves, all the while trying to keep up with our scattered offspring, who have their own situations to ponder.

I suspect that we are in the midst of middle-age crazy. We're too old and have too many considerations to wander aimlessly for long. We are too young to give up on creating new goals, both for career and for our personal lives. In all the commotion rattling through our brains, one thing remains constant. At the core, we have each other.

Jim runs his hand along my thigh and kisses the back of my neck, sending a chill down my spine. Dim the lights and cue the music. Sometimes I am a morning person. Very much so.

CHAPTER 20
Conversations Over Dinner

Jim lifts his glass of Cabernet and watches as I finish the last of my roasted chicken and brown rice. As always, he finishes well ahead of me and nurses his wine to keep me company until I'm done.

A classic rock station plays in the background and Jim is rhythmically strumming his fingers in time with the beat. Smokey and Bandit are prancing in the sunny bay window beside us, vainly attempting to engage the birds as they flit past.

I am chatting away, bouncing from movies to family to my morning at work. Jim doesn't mind this type of chatter, because he knows it indicates that I'm feeling well.

I finish up my wine and blow out the single candle. "What are you thinking about?" I ask.

"Warthogs."

Mutual laughter. We use that word when we mean to say, "not much of anything in particular." We got it from a decades-old episode of *Saturday Night Live* that stuck in my head lo these many years.

"How would you like to start a blog?" I knew Jim had a train of thought going there. Sometimes when he's contemplating something, I can almost see the wheels spinning inside his head.

I've only recently figured out what the word blog even means and can't help laughing at the prospect of actually publishing something online. I've always been a rather private person, with a streak of shyness to boot. He knew that I'd been doing some writing and that I seemed to be enjoying it.

"Sounds like a great idea ... we could blog about what we talked about at dinner!" Suddenly the concept seems like fun. We both like to write and what could be better than a hobby we can share together?

Our small home office is where he spends most of his time and I love being in there while he works. Even when he's preoccupied with a web design project, he occasionally stops to point something out to me or ask my opinion.

The blog would give me the opportunity to be more involved in the online world that is such a big part of Jim's life. The very thing that attracted me to him in the first place was his talent with the written word. For awhile, we played around with writing a story together, each writing a paragraph and handing it back to the other. It was a wonderful exercise but, naturally, our story sounded as though two people were writing it. It was fun while it lasted. This could be just the thing to liven things up.

As we clear the table, we discuss it further. The plan is that Jim will set up two blogs, one for each of us. We will individually write our own version of our dinner conversation without collaboration and end up with a he said/she said blog that will probably be read by no one but ourselves.

Jim wipes off the old kitchen table and gently kisses me before heading back down the hall to the office to finish up some work. The wine has gone to my head a bit and, despite my inability to carry a tune, I sing along, rather loudly, with the soulful music as I wash the dishes. *"Me and Mrs. Jones ..."*

The next day, we have a blog called Conversations Over Dinner. It is a goofy concept, done for our own enjoyment and for laughs, so we are hesitant to use our real names. If we use pseudonyms, we will be able to speak more freely, but Jim will also have to cover our tracks so that we are not easily traceable.

"I think we should take names that begin with the same letter as our real names," I said. "I think I'll be Amanda."

"If your name was Amanda, I'd probably call you Mandy. I'll be Jake." Thus, Jake and Mandy are born and tentatively write their first posts about life around their dinner table. It is oddly satisfying, this co-writing thing. Within a week or so, I am loving it and thinking about tackling the more serious topic of multiple sclerosis, though it won't necessarily fit in with our Conversations Over Dinner theme. I want it to be more serious, something to help people with MS share information and offer support to each other. Little do I realize just how many MS blogs there are in the world. If I knew then I probably would have run screaming for the hills.

Jim creates a second blog for me and we call it MS Maze (www.msmaze.com). Brand new to the blogosphere, here I am now working on two blogs and realizing, once again, just how much I enjoy writing.

Through MS Maze, I begin to connect with other people who have MS. We share our experiences and learn from each other.

Barely seven weeks into the blog experiment, I return from work to find an intriguing email waiting for me. It is not lost on us that we seem to receive a lot of news – both good and bad – through email.

This one is from a producer at The Health Central Network who is searching for bloggers to contribute to the MS section and, based on my writing on MS Maze, I am being invited to join the team. Thinking it very well could be a scam, I do some online sleuthing, then ask Jim to do the same. It is, indeed, the real deal.

They want me to share my personal stories and insights with their readers … and they want to pay me for it. It is an honor to be asked and after a week of back and forth, a contract is signed. Because my online persona is already linked to Mandy, I decided to stick with that. My photo is overlaid with a green mask so that only my eyes peek out.

So Mandy Crest begins writing twice a week for Multiple Sclerosis Central, sharing personal observations about living life with a chronic disease. Now a partner in WebCamp One, LLC, my writing is beginning to produce a modest income.

In short order, my incoming email is filled with introductions by people from all over the world who have MS, people who appreciate my articles and want to share their stories with me. My world is widening.

MS is again the number one topic in our home, but in a very different way. Now it's about something bigger than ourselves. It's about reaching out into a world beyond the walls of our own home.

Up to now, Jim and I felt fairly alone in our experiences with MS. Suddenly we find ourselves commiserating with strangers and finding out that our situation is not unique. The feelings we have, the frustrations, and the epiphanies are not ours alone. There are more of us, more souls who are bound together by a common thread.

Before long, I am pitching an idea to the site producer. How about a spouse/caregiver perspective? Another contract came our way and soon Jake is weighing in on the caregiver side. Jake and Mandy Crest have become our public faces, our alter egos. It is as if there are two couples living in our home.

One afternoon, while perusing the web, I stumble across a blog called Women Over 40 Rock! It is an engaging look at women in Hollywood and how their careers often come to screeching halt upon reaching their 40th birthday. The blog posts were few and far between, though, so I dig a little deeper. The blog is published by a group of ladies known as In The Trenches Productions (ITTP). They know first hand how Hollywood works – and they aim to change all that.

In the persona of Mandy, I feel confident enough to approach the owners of the blog and offer my writing services. The email goes to a standard info@ address, so I really don't know who will be on the receiving end. I introduce myself as a woman over 40 who can help them keep their blog content fresh and help them raise their online profile through blog listing directories and social networking.

The reply comes from Debbie Zipp, a veteran Hollywood actress who played a wide variety of roles, most notably in the recurring role of Donna on *Murder She Wrote*. She is interested, but expresses doubt about a long-term agreement. She suggests a three-month trial. The other women behind In The Trenches Productions are Judith Drake, Jan Bina, and Claire Callaway.

Still hiding behind Mandy, I write my first piece for Women Over 40 Rock and title it "Our Time is Now." Just to make sure that I won't embarrass myself, I ask Jim to take a look at it before submitting it to Debbie. His edits are just what it needs to give it that little something extra, and it is an instant hit with Debbie. She is thrilled that I captured the spirit of what ITTP is trying to do. It is the beginning of a long-term gig and enormously supportive new relationships. Because we live on opposite coasts, I've never met the ladies of ITTP, but nevertheless count them among my friends.

Jim is beside himself with happiness for me, proud of what I managed to do in such a short time. With his wonderful editorial skills, we are quite a team. It suddenly dawns on me that this is precisely what he had in mind when he brought up the idea of blogging. He saw a glimmer of something in me and nurtured it, just to see if it would blossom. He knew I would never have taken that first step without a nudge … so he nudged. I love this man. "You know you're a freelance writer, right?"

Me? A freelance writer? I suppose I am. I've got two paying clients, two steady gigs. This is really something. I wonder just how far I'll be able to take this. Is this what I've been searching for? Could I possibly become one of those people who successfully meld hobby and career?

CHAPTER 21
Bad Day to be Man of the House

Today is primary day. Here in Virginia Super Tuesday is behind us and precious few candidates from either party remain standing. Our country is in crisis on many fronts and health care reform is constantly on our minds. For that reason we feel compelled to make an extra effort to do our part today.

It's a very cold, gray day and I am deep in the throes of a major relapse, making walking or standing an exhausting chore and my arms straining to the very limit. I didn't go to work today because I failed the infamous blow dryer test.

To add to the day's commotion, Bandit suddenly became very ill and Jim had to take him to the veterinarian. The news wasn't good and we fear his life is hanging in the balance as we head off to the polls. Thankfully, the voting line is short. I'm shivering and Jim has to steady me, but we manage to cast our ballots.

Back at home, we each settle in at our computers. Just before 5:00 p.m., the phone rings, the caller I.D. identifying the animal hospital. We make eye contact, instinctively knowing what the ringing phone means. Our beloved Bandit, our big "galumph," just five years old, succumbed to a bladder blockage that shut down his kidneys within 24 hours of the first symptom. We hug and cry at our loss, then turn our thoughts to Smokey. Her world is about to be turned upside down.

It is one of those days when being the man of the family is not an easy role. Because I am having such a rough time of it physically, Jim sets off alone to the animal hospital to retrieve Bandit's remains. I watch as he drives away, this dark and bleak day getting worse by the minute.

When he returns, we each hold Bandit for a moment, then prepare him for burial. Poor Jim! The ground is frozen and it takes him three tries to find a spot soft enough for the grave. I watch from inside, crying and feeling utterly useless. I should be out there helping, but there is nothing I can do. Jim is on his own.

Blubbering, I pick up the phone and call Tommy. "Bandit died." I'm not sure why I chose to call him at this moment except that he's such a kind soul and I knew he would comfort me.

I knew Tommy had a kind spirit from the moment he was born and first placed in my arms. It just radiated off him. Even before his first birthday, he had mastered the art of the hug. He was the only baby I ever knew who would pat me on the back when we hugged. We called that the "tappy hug." Yes, we named his various hugs. There was also a "squeezey hug," and a "gentle hug." These days we have an "email hug," and the "phone hug," and that's what I needed today. He didn't let me down.

Bandit was laid to rest with his favorite blue ball beside an evergreen in the middle of our large backyard. Good-bye, our big galumph.

It was five years ago when we showed up at an animal shelter to find a cat. We did so because we felt our home was too clean and too lacking in chaos. As soon as we laid eyes on him, we knew he was ours. One of a litter of five, he was entangled in a ball of black fur, which turned out to be three of his siblings. We took turns holding him to make sure that we were a good fit. We both felt an immediate bond with our new friend.

Even though we already made our choice, we couldn't help noticing that there was another kitten from the same litter, nervously sitting by herself in a corner of the cage. We felt strangely attracted by her tentative demeanor, so we decided to get to know her as well. We were officially in love – times two!

Bandit quickly took the dominant position to Smokey's submissive, yet very feisty role. They grew big – Bandit weighing in at 18 pounds and Smokey at 12, but there wasn't an ounce of fat on either one of them, they were just big, beautiful animals. If you happened to catch Bandit out of the corner of your eye, you might mistake him for a small dog. We received many compliments about his amazing natural beauty. Gorgeous he was, but one would never accuse him of being graceful, hence the name "galumph." He never seemed to grasp the reality of his own size, and therefore gave us plenty of laughs.

The duo more than fulfilled their duties as keepers of chaos. Their playing and chasing games sounded like a herd of wildebeest. Cat hair and commotion entered the neat and tidy interior of our home. Bandit was the town crier, always making noise of some kind or another. An unusual cat, he would spend hours nestled in Jim's arm, positioned like an infant, while we watched television at night. We never regretted our decision to bring these two lovable pals home.

With Bandit's sudden departure from this world, Smokey is already displaying signs of loss, sitting in one spot for hours on end and eating little. The rest of the time she spends vainly meowing and searching for her lifelong companion. We worry about her wellbeing and consider acquiring a new kitten to take her mind of her troubles, but it is too soon to think about that. When Bandit left, the chaos seemed to go with him.

A few weeks later, Smokey is beginning to adjust to her new life in a single-cat home. She is increasingly vocal and adventurous. We begin to realize just how dominant Bandit had been, and that her less sociable behavior was a result of her place in the family hierarchy.

With newfound confidence, Smokey has become a very active member of our little household. Chaos has returned, thanks to the newly crowned queen of the manor.

Bandit will always be with us in spirit. I still picture our big galumph, patrolling the house and checking in on his sister. Meanwhile, Smokey carries on, doing double duty, as the keeper of chaos. She even took over Bandit's spot on Jim's lap each night as we watch television.

CHAPTER 22
Don't We Take Care of These People?

My first visit with a new neurologist means that he wants new MRI scans. His examination is very thorough, he gives us more time for questions and answers than most, and we feel very comfortable with him. He orders an MRI of the brain, neck, and spine, both with and without contrast.

A month later, we are stunned to find that the total cost of the tests come to $10,000 and our out-of-pocket expense is $3,000. That doesn't include the doctor's visits or the fees for the doctors who read the scans. The interpretation of the results took about 30 seconds. No change, nothing remarkable to report.

Sure, we're very pleased that I am not riddled with new lesions, but dazed and confused by the charges. In the past several years, we've gone from bad to worse with health care expenses, with no end in sight. It is taking a toll. We are keenly aware that a crisis is looming. In my years of comfortable ignorance, I never saw this coming.

Months ago we tried to get the ball rolling on finding health insurance options for when my COBRA coverage period ends, but could not get insurers to speak to us about it. They insist that you wait until you are in your last month before they will offer a quote. The stress level was ratcheted up a notch as we waited and worked on getting quotes. It's pretty hard to plan financially for something if you don't have numbers to work with.

Back in the early 90's, when President Clinton took on the whole health care issue, I was still a fairly healthy young woman with a fantastic group insurance policy. Back then I even had the privilege of vision and dental coverage. I didn't have to think about it as a personal issue because it had never been a problem for me and I didn't see why it should be.

Don't all working people have insurance? Still, I had a great deal of compassion for the working poor and people who did not have the protections that I enjoyed. I didn't think it was right for anyone in America to go without something so basic to life. But didn't we take care of such people anyway? Weren't there programs of some sort? If there weren't, then it certainly ought to be fixed. I was for reform, but it wasn't personal. Yet.

We knew that finding health insurance with MS wouldn't be a walk in the park, but we are devastated by the outright rejection and lack of options. When dealing with potential insurers, MS is a real conversation killer. MS? Okay, move along, nothing more to see here.

I feel it in an intensely personal way, abandoned by a system that seems intent on punishing me for actually needing health care. A mini depression is settling over me as I realize how profoundly this will affect our finances, not just now, but forever and not just for us, but for our families. Because of me, everything we've managed to build throughout our whole lives is on the line. Everything we wanted to do for our children will have to be reevaluated as well.

In Virginia, state law allows insurers to reject applicants with a pre-existing condition, and they didn't hesitate for a moment. There is only one company that MUST offer some type of policy, but they get to decide what to offer and the law sets no caps on premiums they may charge. There is no high-risk pool, no other protections for people like us. That's how I ended up with an expensive policy with a $5,000 deductible for major medical, $5,000 for prescription medications, and $10,000 for tier 4 drugs. Naturally, multiple sclerosis injectables are tier 4 drugs. In addition to my high premiums, that means my co-pay for my MS medication is now $500 per month.

Jim, being a freelancer, also carries an individual policy, although his is less expensive and covers much more than mine. Together, our medical expenses each month are more than our mortgage – and that's if we don't actually use it.

Health care reform is suddenly becoming a very real and oh, so personal topic in our home. I begin writing about it and educating myself on the facts. I can see the future and it doesn't look good. If it is true for me, it is true for millions of others. It's not only about the uninsured. It's about the under-insured. It's about people who are dropped from their policies when they are diagnosed with cancer or some other expensive disease. It's about a country that casts aside the ill. The very idea of it weighs so heavily on me that I can no longer go a single day without thoughts of health care taking up space in my brain.

I know life isn't fair. Some people get sick, some don't. Some people die young, some live to a ripe old age. It's all in the cards you're dealt and to equate good health with fairness would be a terrible mistake. Working in a funeral home has definitely put that in perspective. But health care itself? Certainly, in a country as rich as ours, we can find a way to take care of our own. If nothing else, to enact laws that protect individuals from being kicked when they're down, to offer some alternatives other than being subjected to the whims of a single insurance company. There is a lot of talk about freedom of choice ... but choice is something that I no longer have. I can't choose another insurance plan. I can't choose to relocate, since in most U.S. states I am completely uninsurable. I do not have freedom of choice and I deeply resent it.

Health insurance tied to employment is crippling us all. It makes no sense that upon losing a job you also lose your health insurance. After losing both, how many people are in a position to afford COBRA? No matter what anybody claims, losing health insurance is pretty much losing access to ongoing health care. I am insured and I've been rejected by doctors simply because they didn't like the particular insurance policy I have!

It just galls me that I've played by the rules all these years. I've had health insurance since I was 18 years old and had my first full-time job. No insurer ever gave me a refund because I was healthy. Now that I need health care, I am persona non grata.

I am pouring my thoughts into blog posts, speaking from the heart about what I, and millions of people like me, are experiencing. We want nothing more than a fair shake.

Writing is now a big part of my daily routine. My blogs, Conversations Over Dinner and MS Maze, are a garden that must be tended to each day in order to flourish. My work with The Health Central Network and In the Trenches Productions adds to my responsibilities. I no longer feel like a part-time worker, but a person with two part-time jobs. How about that?

Lying around on the sofa watching mindless television is no longer a daily activity. Good riddance, channel surfing days. Hello, trusty laptop.

A pattern is definitely forming in that I often receive big news via email. Today's email is from an editor at *MSFocus*, a magazine produced by the Multiple Sclerosis Foundation. She read a post I wrote for MS Maze that spoke to the issue of skyrocketing medical costs and wanted to know if I would write an article for publication in *MSFocus*, one that would put hard numbers to paper.

I was thrilled at the opportunity, but somewhat hesitant. When I explained my use of a pen name to the editor, she gave the impression that my real name would be her preference. Where am I going with this writing thing, anyway? It seemed like a good idea when writing the personal blogs, to keep my identity private, but I'm beginning to question the wisdom of that decision going forward. After discussing it with Jim, we made the decision to use my real name.

I thoroughly enjoyed the process of working with the editor, meeting her needs while voicing my own concerns about the state of health care, particularly for MS patients.

The article was titled, "The Financial Reality of Multiple Sclerosis" and listed our actual payments for premiums, co-pays, deductibles, and the facts of life about MS medications.

I wrote about my now all too familiar story – how when my MS symptoms first appeared, I held a full-time job that provided me with good insurance, and how by the time my MS was diagnosed, the severity of my symptoms forced me into a part-time job with no group insurance coverage. I wrote that with Jim and I both having individual insurance, our absolute minimum monthly health care costs were $1,339, providing that during that month we did not actually use any health care. Little did I know at the time how rapidly that absolute minimum would accelerate – to the tune of around 30 percent annually – as would our anxiety. A scant two years later, I would look back upon these figures as a bargain. The enormity of the yearly increases would take a tremendous toll in the years to come.

I am fairly certain that if drastic changes are not made, I will not make it to Medicare age without falling off the insurance rolls. No insurance and no medication to continue fighting MS, not to mention any other health concerns that arise. It's a simple fact of dollars and cents. We are in an insurance death spiral.

It was a joy to see my name – my real name – in a print magazine. I am a writer. I now identify myself that way and believe it to be true. It is giving me a new sense of purpose.

Another day, another email. This one, addressed to Mandy, comes from a reporter with *The Washington Post*. She read an article I wrote for The Health Central Network titled, "Wall Street, Main Street, and MS," in which I speak of the enormity of the health care situation as it relates to the overall economy, and the impact on people who have been diagnosed with chronic illness, and she wanted to speak with me on the subject.

Despite my newfound confidence in writing, I have no such confidence in my speaking ability. Nevertheless, I am intrigued and arrange to speak with her.

The resulting article, "As Budgets Tighten, More People Decide Medical Care Can Wait," spoke about people putting off medical tests and procedures, or doing without medications because of the cost. It is shocking to see my name – my real name – used in an article about access to health care. It is troubling to realize that getting sick can quickly spiral a family into a world of financial trouble, where the possibility of losing everything suddenly becomes a reality. So many people in crisis. The article is spread far and wide and for the first time I am the subject of heated comments. Some people come right out and call me a liar. They don't believe that an MRI costs that much or that my out-of-pocket for the procedure was that high. They fail to understand the system of health insurance and differences from state to state and from policy to policy, especially in the individual market. Who knows what an MRI costs, anyway? What you pay is not necessarily what I pay. It costs what they say it costs. Period.

Other folks say it was my responsibility to shop around for a better MRI deal or a better insurance policy, but where you live has a great deal to do with your ability to shop around. Misguided people everywhere want to point the finger at me. As long as it's my own fault, they can rest easy at night, knowing they are safe. But there are also many, many people who get it, based on their own personal experiences.

Always an intensely private person, these two national mentions of my name came at the perfect intersection of ideas. Stay the course as an anonymous blogger, or come out from the shadows and take a shot. It's not a minor decision. In the persona of Mandy, I am free to speak without repercussions, but unable to use identifying information. I can shield myself from the negativity.

As Ann, I have a lot at stake. My reputation and that of my family is on the line.

Jim and I talk it over at length and decide that if I want to take my freelance writing to another level, and if I want to become a voice in the health care debates, my best bet is to use my own name. It's a big step. Up to this point, we've managed to keep Jake and Mandy fairly separate from Jim and Ann. Outing me would also out him. The online world lends itself to links and various networking sites that I will be able to make better use of under my own name. It is both exciting and quite intimidating.

I'm wearing several hats now. I'm a correspondence secretary in a funeral home, who also happens to assist in her bosses' aircraft salvage business. Selling airplane parts from an office in a funeral home is, I suspect, a bit unusual. I am also a blogger and freelance writer. I am a multiple sclerosis patient advocate and another voice in the chorus for health care reform. Of those, finding my way as a writer has taken center stage. I know in my heart that this is the illusive "thing" I have been searching for, and so does Jim.

Trying to grow a freelance writing career without a website is a difficult task. Editors and publishers don't have a lot of time to spare when looking for a writer. Having all your information and samples of your work all in one place is essential.

Once I came to this realization, I asked Jim what he thought about creating such a website for me. I knew the site should include a portfolio, contact information, and – fingers crossed – testimonials. With little input from me, Jim managed to capture my personality and style, creating a beautiful, elegantly simple website that would serve as my face to the world.

He created the feel I wanted, using colors and style that fit my personality, even managing to include a photo of Smokey and Bandit on the home page.

With the main framework in place, he used a content management system that would allow me to periodically make changes and update a blog without his assistance. With the debut of AnnPietrangelo.com, Ann and Mandy are publicly joined at last.

I've been devouring books about freelancing and writing, learning how to pitch stories, find jobs, and build a portfolio. My daily "to do" list now includes searching for additional writing jobs. For the first time in a long while, I feel enthusiastic and, dare I say, energetic. Not steroid energetic, but naturally energetic.

Jim is very fond of a quote by William Arthur Ward, the American author, editor, pastor, and teacher. "If you can imagine it, you can achieve it. If you can dream it, you can become it." I'm becoming rather fond of the quote myself. I am imagining it; I am dreaming it. I'm already becoming it; I will achieve it. Writing is no longer just a silly notion, but what I think about during every free moment.

I finally figured out what I'm going to be when I grow up.

Ann Pietrangelo

CHAPTER 23
You Don't Belong Here

Where is this place? I am lost beyond all hope. I don't know where I am or where I am going, and there are far too many people around. I am walking, or trying to anyway, but it feels like trying to walk with tree trunks for legs. I want to make use of my cane, but it is only ankle high, too short to be of any help; but now it is too tall. When I ask people for help, they only laugh. "You don't belong here." They prevent me from sitting to rest and refuse to give me directions home. I am so alone and vulnerable.

Dreams are a window into the subconscious, or so they say. I am a very vivid dreamer, and they often stick with me for days, as I try to unravel the meaning behind my nighttime flights of fancy.

Until now, I have been healthy in my dreams, free of any physical constraints of MS or any other ailment, living in worlds of my own making. An alternate reality of my subconscious. My dreams of late have an obvious theme.

In another dream, I was blind and fully aware that it was due to MS. But I didn't see darkness. That's because I was outside myself, observing my own reaction to going blind. I felt empathy toward my other, less fortunate self, yet strangely serene.

A psychologist would have a field day with these dreams, I'm sure, but they are not hard to decipher. Even when I am in remission, thoughts of an MS relapse are with me, even if they are pushed to the farthest reaches of my consciousness.

The dreams serve as a wakeup call; a prompt to search my soul for meaning and purpose.

"You don't belong here," they said. But I do. I do belong here. I finally understand and accept that I do belong. Not to any particular category or group of people, not to any one mindset or circumstance. There is no need to go searching for the right label to pinpoint exactly where it is I belong. I just belong!

I don't like having MS, but as Jim always says, "It is what it is." We're dealing with it and working around the damn thing every which way we can. Life must, and does, go on. I belong.

A lot of things are beginning to fall into place. Jim and I have settled in to married life with ease. In spite of the lingering doubts about our careers, place of residence, and longing for family, we are comfortable as a couple. In the great scheme of things, we've been together only a short period of time, but it is as though we've always been together. I belong.

Ah, midlife. I'm on the high side of my 40's now, and I am coming into my own at long last. My body is not what it used to be and my face is slowly turning into my mother's face. My hands, at times, remind me of my grandmother's hands – at least when the weather is dry and I am in dire need of lotion. But the thing is, I am no longer agonizing about it. Coping with MS has taught me a great many things, one of them being acceptance of what is inevitable – like aging. The alternative, after all, is death, something I am reminded of every day at work.

Older women have always had a hard time in our society. They've lied about their age because they knew that youth was prized and maturity, at least in the female gender, was not. The coming of age of the baby boomer generation is changing all that.

Certainly, a great many women today are learning to embrace their age and the sense of freedom that comes with it. We've earned every darn wrinkle and we're not going to apologize for them.

I don't consider myself beautiful, or even pretty, and have never been accused of being cute. I never fit that cookie-cutter version of ideal female beauty; nevertheless, I know I am attractive. When I look in the mirror, most of the time I like what I see. Sometimes, not so much, especially if MS in on the attack, but that's a different story.

I say forget all the advice of the beauty experts who would hammer away at your self-esteem and tell you how many ways you don't make the cut. Not that I don't take pride in my appearance. I admit to never leaving the house without a bit of makeup, I color my hair and style it every day, at least when MS allows. I file my nails and moisturize my skin. I shave and tweeze and primp. I maintain a suitable weight for my height and build. I want to look my best, and I don't apologize for that, but I'm respectful of Mother Nature and gravity and all that comes with growing older, for time and gravity serve no master.

If I concentrate on nothing but the individual parts that make up the whole, I could make quite a list of my flaws. My nose could be cuter and my thighs just ain't what they used to be, and years of injections have created puckers in my skin, which is a bit too white. It sounds better if I call it porcelain or ivory. And I'm told I've got funny facial expressions, but I am generally unaware of them until someone shrieks.

I am Seinfeld's "two-face" date. Thoroughly fetching in certain light; equally horrifying in other lighting. Once a waitress served my food and recoiled slightly, asking, "What's wrong?"

Puzzled, I answered, "Nothing ..."

"Oh, you made a disgusted face. I thought something was wrong with your food."

Did she say, "disgusted" or "disgusting?"

"I made a disgusting face? I'm sorry, I didn't mean to. Everything is fine." Oh, just kill me now. How is it I so often manage to convey the wrong message with my face? My face should not be allowed to speak for me.

In spite of the flaws, I am most definitely an attractive woman, a confident woman, a woman of substance. Age be damned, I still like the way I look, funny face and all.

I will continue my best to stay healthy and vibrant, but will celebrate rather than run from my age. I've earned my place in this world. The human being who resides within this slightly-less-than-perfect body is thriving, and it shows. I belong.

The creation of my new website worked like hanging out a "freelance writing" shingle. I've picked up some stray writing jobs here and there and gotten quite comfortable referring to myself as a writer. My clients thus far have been very pleased with my work.

The intersection of multiple sclerosis, marriage, and midlife has been a wild ride, that's for sure, but I am in full bloom.

CHAPTER 24
Is That a Smudge on Your Face or Just Your Mascara?

What could be more traditional than Thanksgiving in New England? The long drive during the holidays is not exactly our idea of a good time, but the destination and the Thanksgiving holiday are well worth the effort.

We only get up to Rhode Island about once a year, generally for Thanksgiving, which is usually hosted by my niece and her husband, or by my nephew. This year is Nephew's turn and the whole gang will be in attendance, including his fiancé; my niece, her husband, and their two little girls; another niece and her boyfriend; and Mom. Then there's Sis and my eldest brother, who tragically lost his wife a few years ago, along with his companion ... and his ex-wife who happens to be the mother of my nephew and one of my nieces. Although we grew up together and never used the term, my eldest brother and Sis are really my half-siblings, so their father and his wife are also in attendance. Then there's Jim and me. Talk about an eclectic group! A true modern family.

Those present remember the loved ones who are unable to be with us today, and those who have passed on.

David, Liz, and Tommy are spending Thanksgiving with their father in Illinois. We visit New Jersey to spend time with Jim's family several times every year because it is a substantially shorter drive than the trip to New England. We don't get to see his daughter in New Orleans as often and I haven't seen my two Texas-based brothers in years.

So we have plenty of family, but we are not present in their lives for the most part, nor are they in ours, outside of our thoughts. There is a certain sense of separateness that stays with Jim and me, whether we are at home in Virginia, or sitting around breaking bread with family. We are strangely detached from our elders, our siblings, and even our children.

As we gather around the Thanksgiving table and all its bounty, much attention is lavished on the young girls and laughter fills the air. They've got some inside jokes that Jim and I don't share, and although we are all family, we are guests in this home and, in a strange way, guests in the family. In spite of that separateness, we are having a marvelous time, goofing on each other, sipping wine, and talking up a storm.

I'm in pretty good shape right now, not currently using a cane, but by day's end I'm exhausted and happy to lay my head on the pillow. It is unseasonably cold, and the wind is howling outside the window as we fade off into slumber.

The next day, my sister tells me that she has some brand new shoes that don't fit properly, and would be mine for the taking. After trying on several pairs of her shoes, I pack up two pairs, plus a necklace and earrings she no longer wants. It's been decades since I've received hand-me-downs from Sis, and I'm thrilled – both because I have some great new things, and because it feels almost as though I'm taking a part of her home with me. Indeed, I will be thinking of her when I wear her things.

Sis and I were not particularly close as children, but we were almost always in close proximity. We had to share a bedroom in a small home with three brothers, two parents, and one bathroom. You get the idea.

Before we managed to score twin beds, we even had to share a sleep sofa. That kind of forced togetherness would test any sibling relationship. Despite the trivial trials and tribulations, ours managed to survive.

I secretly liked having her next to me at night because I was afraid of the dark. Although she feigned indifference, she habitually gave in to my pleadings and put her arm around me in a protective pose until I fell asleep.

Sis is five years older than I and, when we were little, I envied some of her possessions. Oh, how I wanted to walk in her shoes! Literally. In the third grade, I was particularly fond of her winter boots. They were black with fur at the top, and went to mid-calf. They were about as close to the popular and stylish "go-go boots" of the time as I ever hoped to get. My goal was to be "cool," but I was always slightly off the mark.

Mom was still insisting that I wear my little red rubber snow boots that fit over my shoes, despite my protests that not a single other girl in my class still wore these ugly baby boots. Sis's boots were getting a little tight on her feet and I wanted them – badly. When Sis finally had enough of the tight boots, Mom reluctantly turned them over to me, even though they were still way too big for my feet. Nevertheless, I proudly clumped off to school in them. I sort of feel that way today, whenever I slip into my big sister's shoes.

Every time we visit Rhode Island, there is some silly little item that brings back a flood of memories. This time it's a mint condition Hamilton Beach milk shake machine, circa 1950, residing in a place of honor in Sis's kitchen. It's about as close as we come to having a family heirloom. I'm fairly convinced that she thought I'd come unglued when I requested that she remove it from its perch so I could photograph it, but she humored me anyway. It's something big sisters instinctively do.

Whenever I see the milk shake machine with its funky jadeite color, smooth lines, and gleaming metal, I am instantly transported back to the era of my youth.

When we were kids, the good old Hamilton Beach was stashed away in a kitchen cupboard, never seeing the light of day until called into duty. It rarely made an appearance outside of Christmas when Dad – who wasn't exactly known for his social skills or his kitchen abilities – would offer up a strange concoction of eggs, sugar, and … I'm not sure I want to know what else … and called it egg nog. We had a ball watching him work what we thought was magic, highlighted by the *whirrrrrr* of the Hamilton Beach mixer. It was a comforting sound. Actually drinking the stuff was secondary.

The only other "recipe" of Dad's was a weird salad dressing that he called "slop," something that made Mom wince. Naturally, that made it even more appealing. My brother tells tales of a "rubber guts cake" incident, another kitchen horror, which I do not recall, although I do recall the brotherly caper that ended with "cantaloupe innards" being unceremoniously dumped on my long hair, but I digress.

It's funny, the memories that come flooding back at the sight of a kitchen appliance. I suppose it's because the kitchen truly is the heart of the home, and the memories made there are the most comforting. Thanks for the memories, Sis.

For dinner, my nephew asked if there was a particular restaurant we'd like to visit or if we'd prefer to stay home for a game/pizza party night. No contest. Roll out the dough and break out the Boggle, because this family time is the reason for our visit.

He has a large, gorgeous kitchen, with modern stainless appliances and granite counter tops. He and his fiancé are obviously enjoying the process of preparing pizza dough and cutting the veggies and toppings, spreading it all on the counter in a do-it-yourself fashion. There are plenty of giggles as we line up to make our individual pizzas.

After we're all appropriately stuffed, Jim and I get our first look at a game of Wii, and it's pretty obvious that we're going to want one of our own in the very near future, with our very own little Mii characters.

"Hey, Bug, do you play Boggle?" My brother is the only person on the planet who calls me "Bug." I was born tiny – under five pounds. Apparently, I was such a cute little thing that someone decided I was "cute as a ladybug." I'm told I was called that for awhile, but as I grew the name fell by the wayside. With everyone but big brother. He shortened it to Bug and continues to carry on the tradition to this day.

Group photos, some more wine, a crazy game of Boggle, and time for a bathroom break.

While washing my hands, I take a moment to check out my face in the mirror. Lovely. I have a giant black smudge over my right eye, just below the eyebrow. And we've been posing for photos all night! I leave the bathroom and tell Jim, "Would you believe I've had this big black smudge over my eye all night?"

"I didn't notice," he said.

You've got to be kidding me. It was a giant black smudge right over my eye!

"I saw it, but I didn't say anything," says my brother.

"I noticed it, too," chimes in Sis. "I thought it was makeup."

Oh, that's a good one. Actually, it was smudged mascara. Surely no one thought I put it there as a fashion statement.

"Well, I wasn't sure what it was," says my niece.

Oh, yeah. *That's* what family is all about! I miss that. No ... I really do.

Ann Pietrangelo

CHAPTER 25
Blogging for Health Care

"Welcome to the Care2 blogging team! We are delighted to have you on board for the Health Policy channel."

Who, me? This is good news. Care2 is an enormously popular site around the world, a leader in green issues, and has recently launched several "cause" channels, one being health policy. I'm thrilled to have made the cut! The sample I submitted centered on the great need for comprehensive health care reform. It was a passionate plea, from a very personal perspective.

My views on health care in the United States and around the world will now be read on a regular basis. This is an opportunity to bump it up a notch, to improve not only my writing, but my ability to speak intelligently to the issues and to engage readers in an exchange of ideas.

For the most part, it is an uplifting experience, but I am once again taken aback by some of the comments of the blogosphere. While the vast majority are insightful, uplifting, or interesting, some are just mean spirited. I try not to take it personally or to be overly sensitive, but the Internet lends itself to this kind of thing. It gives people the confidence to say things they would never say in person.

I'm learning that sometimes, comments have nothing whatsoever to do with me or with what I write. Apparently, some folks troll the Internet trying to spread a particular agenda regardless of where they post it. I've even seen ads for commenters posted on writing job boards. My skin is going to have to get a bit thicker to withstand this and still speak my mind about health reform.

The supportive comments and emails more than outweigh the bad and I feel good about what I'm contributing.

I'm learning to be a lot more careful with my words, trying to imagine how they would be read by someone else. I may write them in my voice, but the interpretation is up to the reader. Now that I think about it, I was in the fifth grade when I first learned how a single word can change the entire meaning of a sentence.

We were assigned the task of writing a one-page description of ourselves, both our physical attributes and our personality traits. The teacher planned to read them aloud to the class and we were to guess the author. The purpose, I now know, was to teach us descriptive writing. Fifth grade is a risky time for such an assignment. For one boy, it proved to be very embarrassing.

It was the late sixties, when long hair for young males was very popular. Boys who wanted to be "cool" had longer hair. This particular boy described himself as having "pretty long" black hair. The guessing began with girl names. In fact, no one guessed a boy. That's because the teacher, being a woman, read the sentence emphasizing the word "pretty." Pretty was read in a way that would describe a female attribute. Long was read in an elongated fashion. We were looking for a classmate with pretty, long black hair.

When his name was revealed, the flustered boy vainly tried to explain that he meant "pretty long," as in "fairly long." It was too late; the damage was done. He spent the rest of the year as the boy with the pretty, long black hair. Ouch.

Lesson learned. People don't necessarily read things the way you meant them, and I would be wise to keep that in mind as I choose words for my blog postings.

The more I delve into the topic of health care reform, the more I understand how grave the situation is for the tens of millions of us who have no health insurance and millions more who are underinsured. Lack of health insurance, in many cases, translates into lack of access to health care. It's a matter of life and death and we're letting it happen. I don't know what it's going to take for reform to even begin. I don't understand the reluctance to work on repairing an obviously broken system.

A few years ago, for one of the AMOA's mid-year board meetings, Jim and I traveled to Cabo San Lucas, Mexico. The day before we left on our trip, Jim had been working outside in some shrubbery. The morning of our departure, he noticed that his finger was bothering him somewhat, but decided to ignore it, figuring it would take care of itself. It didn't. Arriving at our hotel, it was now obvious to us that the middle finger of his right hand had an infection of some sort. We thought that maybe he'd been bitten by something or pricked by a rose thorn. In any case, the finger was swelling big time, taking on a rather bulbous look. So much for the golf game he had planned to play the next day.

With the infection getting worse, we were both beginning to worry; our concern for his finger compounded by the fact that we were in Mexico. Would we be able to see a doctor? Would his insurance cover it? Would he get good care?

We began by calling the hotel information desk. It turned out that they had a hotel doctor on call day or night. We explained the situation and were told that the doctor would soon be knocking on our hotel room door. We looked at each other in disbelief. A doctor is going to make a house call to the hotel? Here? Now? We'll believe it when we see it.

And see it we did. Within half an hour the doctor arrived, little black bag and all. Jim managed to smile through the pain ... the doctor was gorgeous! She sat at the little round table and took a look at Jim's finger,

167

which was, unbelievably, still increasing in size. She wasn't sure what caused it, but decided that it needed to be lanced. Pulling the necessary tools out of her bag, she got to work right away. We inquired about cost, but she wasn't particularly interested in speaking of money or insurance. Rather, she seemed genuinely concerned about the finger. Sure, we thought, this is going to cost us big time. We kept quiet though, since we were in no position to push the issue. After all, we clearly needed her help and cost, at that time, was the least of our concerns.

Finishing up, she bandaged Jim's finger and said that she would return the next day to follow up and see if the swelling went down. She left her card and told us to call if it began to look worse. We couldn't believe it. Not only did she come to us and treat Jim on the spot, but she was going to come back and even promised to take our call if there was a problem in between those two visits!

With his middle finger bandaged to high heaven and sticking straight out, Jim quickly attracted his fair share of attention and smiled good-naturedly as the jokes were thrown his way.

But the fickle finger of fate was not to be kind that day. By morning, his finger was swollen even worse than before, and was beginning to cause him a lot of pain. Jim made a call to "his" doctor and told her about the problem.

A few minutes later, we were with the doctor in her office on the hotel grounds. Looking at the finger, she said that she didn't like what was happening. She felt that it needed to be operated on right away. We looked at each other. Operated on! In Mexico! Olé, what a mess.

Picking up the phone, she called a surgeon that she knew whose office was not far from the hotel. Hanging up, we seriously wondered what alternate universe we had stumbled into as she informed us that the surgeon was on his way to the hotel. He would rush over from across town and be with us soon. Having come from a world where I had to wait four to six weeks to see a surgeon in his office, we didn't quite know what to make of this strange turn of events.

Twenty minutes later, the surgeon walked in and quickly got to work on what we now just called "the finger." Like the first doctor, he too told us not to worry about money. We'd work that out later. Jim asked me to leave the room while they worked. He doesn't like being a patient and certainly doesn't like me to witness such things.

Less than 30 minutes later, the doctors were finished. They ordered some antibiotics and gave us instructions about how to care for the finger and warnings about things to look for that might be signs of trouble. Oddly enough, they waited for us to bring up the subject of payment. The doctor then proceeded to tally up the numbers and handed over a bill for $300.00.

We were stunned. Not only did a doctor and a surgeon go out of their way to accommodate us, but they were professional, competent, and extremely friendly. Knowing what medical services cost in the states, we would not have been shocked had the price been 10 times as much. Jim was so amazed and appreciative that he gave them extra. I hate to call it a "tip," because who ever heard of tipping a doctor? It just isn't done. In this case, however, seeing that we were in a foreign land and had a bit of a medical emergency, we simply did not expect the response we received, and we were over-the-top grateful.

The remainder of our Cabo trip was relaxing and wonderful. When we returned home, a follow-up visit to our own physician confirmed a job well done. It may seem like a small thing, but our memories of our Cabo trip always include a hat tip to the doctors on call and our neighbors to the south who treated us so kindly.

I'm not going to be one of those people who constantly talk about the old days and how much better everything was. I understand about selective memory and that times must change. I know that physicians today are faced with a complicated system that doctors of old could never have imagined. These days, your health insurance is the key to your health care.

You can tell a lot about a people by how they treat the ill, and I know we can do better than this. I cannot understand why we allow people to go without medical care, even if it means their death. It is my nature to at least attempt to understand the opposite point of view, but on this I am failing miserably. Blogging for health care is the very least I can do.

CHAPTER 26
I Didn't Think You Noticed Things Like That

"Beep." It's been beeping for two years and we still can't pinpoint it. Our home, like most houses in America these days, is loaded with gadgets and techie things that go beep and boop in the night.

This particular beep is soft and brief and we've given up actually trying to pinpoint its origin. When we're in the office, it seems to be in the room with us, but we've put our ear to every possible device in there to no avail. When we're in the living room, it could just as easily come from downstairs. I once spent 45 minutes sitting in what I figured to be the exact center of the room in my quest for an answer. Nothing. Ah, modern living. Beep.

Technology has it advantages. Wireless Internet access is one of those. We have a very tiny deck outside our kitchen, just large enough for a bistro table, two chairs, and a couple of planters. We've got a bird house and a large bird feeder hanging in the pine trees and Jim keeps our little friends very well fed.

I love taking the laptop and writing out on the deck, surrounded by sunshine, fresh air, and birds. Screaming birds, sometimes. It's spring and they do not approve of my presence out there while they are raising their young families. So instead of the beeping and booping I've got screeching and squawking. Not that I want to get in the way of nature or anything, but I've waited all winter to enjoy the afternoon outdoors in the fresh air.

I move my chair as far from the tree as the tiny deck will allow and resume my writing. Unfortunately for me, these birds have apparently studied Hitchcock's *The Birds* and, after several near misses, one dive-bombs my head. You've made your point, my little feathered friend.

I'd like to work in the office, but lately my animated pecking away at the keyboard has been getting under Jim's skin. He needs to concentrate, to "get in the zone." I consider writing to be a rather quiet, sedentary process, but it seems to be bothering both the birds and my husband. How is it that I'm such a disturbing presence? Go figure. I'm like the man without a country, doomed to wander the high seas, never to have a homeland.

Sometimes I work at the kitchen table in front of the large bay window with the sunshine on my back. When the wooden kitchen chairs start to get to me, I turn to the living room for comfort. Our sofa is just the right marriage between soft and firm, molding to my body as I sink in. The large wooden coffee table is perfect for putting your feet up. That's exactly why we bought it. We specifically chose a sturdy table so that we could put our feet on it without hesitation. I was never one to want furniture that shouldn't be used. Life is way too short for that. This set up is particularly comfortable when in an MS relapse, allowing me to change position often.

Our living room has a unique feature, partly of our own making, partly due to the previous homeowners. They had a large palm tree in a heavy metal pot that they were reluctant to move, so they asked if we wanted it. It was an awfully big pot, so we did some decorating around the palm tree. We added a little ceramic dog, a childhood art project made by Jim's youngest daughter, a couple of small potted plants, and pine cones from the backyard to cover the dirt so the cats wouldn't be tempted to play in it. Then we added a small water fountain with smooth river stones. We have that fountain running from morning until bedtime, every day. There is something supremely soothing about the sound of gently running water. It definitely beats beeping and booping and screeching and squawking. Every time someone enters our home for the first time, this custom-made ensemble becomes a conversation piece. If I can't enjoy the deck and the great outdoors, the living room is a wonderful consolation prize.

Today I'm trying to write an article about multiple sclerosis, but I've received some emails and comments of late that give me pause. I've been called a "beacon," a "hero," and applauded for my wonderfully positive attitude. I'm more than a little uncomfortable with it.

I wonder if, by keeping my worst moments private, I have contributed to the pressure to keep up appearances. By attempting to put my best foot forward, have I wrongfully given the impression that I'm always full of sunshine and roses? I would hate to think that I am contributing to the pressure that the positive attitude police are so successfully foisting on people.

Don't get me wrong. I believe in positive attitude and I believe in a mind/body connection, but I do not believe in magical thinking or that admitting that I'm having a perfectly lousy day is going to unravel my health. Sometimes MS gets to me; sometimes I even indulge in a brief round of self-absorption. It usually occurs on the day that all hell breaks loose and a relapse is going at full throttle, when it takes until lunchtime to shower and dress. Sometimes I even have myself a little cry over it and rather than feeling like failure, it feels like good therapy. It's about losing control over my body.

Because I allow myself that brief period to release the frustration, it generally blows over in a half hour or so. I don't think that makes me a bad person or means that I'm not trying hard enough.

I think the positive attitude patrol functions as a guilt trip in disguise. If you're sick, and you aren't wearing your happy face, you are not doing your duty. But are they really promoting a positive attitude in the best interest of you ... or is it a lopsided attempt to protect themselves from having to deal with your illness or disability? I do not believe that people with health problems have a responsibility to protect people around them from dealing with it.

One of the most frustrating aspects of life with chronic illness is the constant state of flux, and relapsing/remitting MS definitely lives up to its name.

The fact that many of its on-again, off-again symptoms are invisible to observers makes it a particularly difficult series of emotional adjustments, especially if you are prone to worry about what other people think.

It's hard to be taken seriously when people see you looking the very picture of health one day and claiming to be the opposite the next. It probably doesn't help their perceptions when you go to such great lengths to hide the truth.

"I really need to rally because I haven't kept up with the cleaning. There's a lot of cat hair by the front door." Our house features a split foyer with dark hardwood floors, and cat hair seems to congregate by the front door. I've been putting off cleaning it all week, trying to find the energy to even begin to tackle the job of housecleaning.

"Oh, good. I didn't think you noticed things like that."

He said it calmly. He said it without direct accusation. He said it. And it got my hackles up. "What kind of a crack is that?"

"I'm just saying, you don't seem to notice these things. You don't get too wound up about cleaning." And there it is. The whole "but you look so good" phenomenon is instantly crystalized as a case in point. Right here in my own living room. Even the sweetest, most helpful partner in the world is fooled by my outer appearance. He thinks I'm oblivious to the fact that the house needs cleaning?

With all the calm and rationality I can muster, I state my case. "Of course I can see it. I hate it as much as you do. But I get up every morning and force myself to go to work. Then I come home and do my writing. Some days it takes everything I have to put dinner on the table. Just because it doesn't show, doesn't mean that I'm not having trouble, or that I'm not doing everything I can."

I hope that didn't sound as whiny as I think it did. How could he have possibly known? I've gotten very good at the art of planning and plotting to get through the day.

Nobody on the planet has a husband as accommodating as mine. He does more than his share around here and the last thing I want to do is sound as though I am attacking him. Good husband? Yes. Psychic? No.

"I know that. I just hate it." He reaches out to take my hand and I come in for the full cuddle. Damn it! Now I'm going to cry about it? What am I crying about? Well, if that's the way it's going to be, let's just go with it. The tears pour from my eyes and Jim smiles in understanding.

He gets it. I get it. We get it.

Whether it's MS or some other physical challenge, life does not stop to allow us to get a grip. Sometimes life just gets a bit overwhelming. We need not mask legitimate emotions behind a false positive persona.

The trick is not to wallow and let the negatives gain the upper hand, but to deal with them as they occur in order to get to the positive. I really want to make that point in my articles about MS.

I don't want to be seen in a negative light, but as a positive person who lends kinship and support to others through my writing on the subject of MS and chronic illness. On the other hand, the bad days we all experience cannot be avoided. Addressing them openly and honestly doesn't make me a negative person; it makes me human.

As Smokey approaches the trickling water fountain for a drink, I realize just how much I like this room … and this home … and my little job of writing.

Here comes that old positive attitude again. Sometimes I just can't help myself.

CHAPTER 27
The Bocce Balls Don't Get Out Much

I'd just finished with the dinner dishes when David phoned. He said he and a couple of friends are considering a road trip before summer's end, and if they decide to go ahead with it, would we mind at all if they dropped in for a few days? What kind of a crazy question is that? I was positively giddy with excitement.

"When do you think you would be starting out?" Silence. "David … David?"

"Damn! I lost him!"

I hit the call back button, but he's not answering. I repeat the action and wonder what happened when the doorbell rings. Oh, come on.

"Sweetie … could you please get the door? David called and I lost him. I need to get him back on the line … he was talking about visiting soon!"

I hear Jim's footsteps as he makes his way from the office toward the front door. As I dial David's number again, I pace by the front door to see Jim standing there with the door wide open, giving me that lopsided grin of his. Just beyond him stands David, phone in hand and a sly smile. I'll never forget the picture of him standing there like he'd pulled off the surprise of the century. That's exactly what he had done. Several yards behind him are his two friends, kids … well, young men now, whom I've known most of their lives.

I practically fly into David's arms, overjoyed by his surprise. Then I greet Pete and Greg and we troop back into the house. After a 13-hour drive, they are more than eager to relax and enjoy a cool drink.

There had been a few clues that something was up, but I missed them until now. David had led me to believe that with summer classes and his work at a PBS television station, he would be unable to squeeze in a visit for awhile. Lately he had been asking odd questions about our bedtime, any upcoming travel plans, etc. And just a few hours ago I called him but he had abruptly cut me off by saying he just got to work and would have to call me later, if I would be home.

Now he was here, actually here in the flesh! Thankfully, I am in a fairly good remission, so I'll be able to enjoy this visit. They are only staying for a few days and want to get in an afternoon in D.C. before heading to Florida to visit Pat, another childhood pal.

They are a great group of kids, and their childhood antics are as fresh in my mind as if they happened yesterday, but those mischievous little boys grew into great young men. I once towered over them, but I feel so short around these guys now. Not one of them is less than six feet tall. Where did the years go?

Jim excused himself around 11:30 p.m., and Greg and Peter disappeared downstairs, allowing David and me some precious alone time. As usual, we quickly fell into weird reminisces of "the old days." When the kids were little, they enjoyed my own childhood tales. "Tell me about when you were a kid, mommy." Apparently, they will never outgrow this request.

My childhood was fairly dull and left little room for bona fide adventure, but I love to tell stories to children, so my tales revolve around the most mundane of events, and a lot of self-deprecating humor about my childhood missteps.

I was a goofy and naive kid and was always either doing something dumb or falling for someone else's pranks. Like the time I decided, for reasons known only to my youthful self, to put one rock under my sister's bed each day; or how my younger brother and I were so petrified of our family dog that when our errant baseball landed in his territory, one of us had to act as a decoy while the other had the task of retrieving the ball at the risk of losing life and limb. It was a real comedy routine, but the German Shepherd never bit anybody. He was just a lot bigger and louder than us.

I think the success of my storytelling was more about my wild voice and funny facial expressions than anything else. In any case, they still want to hear the same stories and I hope to be telling them to my grandchildren at some point. On the other hand, my kids will probably have their own tales to tell them.

David was a particularly difficult baby and a very hard-to-handle toddler. When he hit three years old, it was like some minor miracle happened. He turned into an angel overnight and finally I could take a deep breath. He's been wonderful ever since.

I was never really certain why he was so ornery, but in the early years it was quite a struggle. When I tried to explain that my child cried all the time and banged his own head against things, people tended to dismiss my frustration as that of first-time mother jitters. "All babies cry," they would say. The kid hardly slept either, but when I tried to tell people, they would scoff. "Babies sleep about 20 hours a day." This one couldn't manage three hours in a row.

He created scenes at the doctor's office, the barbershop, the grocery store ... you name it. The day we were scheduled for an appointment with a pediatric dentist, I finally felt vindicated.

I filled out the forms honestly when asked about behavior. When the dentist called us in to his office, he dismissed me right to my face. "You're just a nervous mother, probably overprotective. He won't be a problem."

I held my tongue, but inside my head, I was screaming. This jerk who had never met me was judging me and I was seething with anger.

A few minutes later, from the waiting room, I heard the commotion begin. Suddenly, I didn't mind that David was a handful. Instead, I was gleeful. I hope he really puts on a show!

Finally, I was called back in. The dentist looked at me sheepishly. "Well, you were right. He doesn't like to be touched ... and he bit my finger pretty good." He held up his finger, now wrapped in gauze. I remained polite, but inside, I was laughing. Thanks, David.

Now there's a story he can tell his own kids someday.

The next afternoon I came home from work at 1:00 and found David, Greg, and Peter in the backyard playing bocce. I stood at the patio door, marveling at the site of this activity in our normally lonely backyard. The bocce balls don't get out much, generally passing for decorative items in a large basket by the fireplace. Today, they are worth their weight in gold. I have an overwhelming sense of contentment.

Only a blink in time earlier, David was the little baby that I vowed to protect and defend from the evils of the world. Things have come full circle. Now he is the one who insists on having an itinerary before I travel, and on hearing his phone ring upon my return. The old parent/child switcheroo is happening much sooner than I expected.

David, when he asks how I am, doesn't always accept "fine" as an answer. "You are? Come on, didn't you say something about your legs giving you a hard time?"

"Well, what I meant was ... relatively fine ... you know, fine for me ... as well as can be expected ... basically really quite very fine ... fabulous indeed." A lot of meaningless words that, when strung together, mean I am touched that you really care about my answer to your "how are you?"

I still have one great big bone to pick with my offspring. Games. They simply cannot deal with me winning anything. To be beaten by Mom – at anything – apparently brands you with a giant LOSER sign across your forehead. "Mom beat you? You must be really bad." Now I do understand how and why this came to be. I've never been the least bit athletic, I don't play many card games, and I don't know much about sports. On the other hand, I'm pretty good competition in word games, completely useless trivia, and now Wii Bowling and Wii Boxing. Really. I can kick major butt in Wii Boxing and, therefore, it is not a cool game to play. Mom might beat you and wouldn't that be embarrassing! Better to just label it a stupid game that you really don't want to play anyway.

Last time David and Tommy were here, I beat them both at Wii boxing and they were absolutely humiliated, laughingly blaming the game and the controller for their losses.

When you win at Wii Boxing, your little Mii character does a little winner dance and I like to dance along. Last time we played, I noticed a camera whirring away and said, "This had better not show up on You Tube!" You guessed it. Somewhere on You Tube is a 15 second clip of me laughing and doing the Mii dance.

Over the next day and a half, we manage some more reminiscing, play cards, share hearty meals, and reconnect. I can't help but shed a few bittersweet tears as I watch the car drive away toward adventure in the sunshine state. They've got so much life ahead of them! They don't know it yet, but they are in the process of making sweet memories for their old age. And David probably has no idea how much happiness his little surprise visit brought us.

Ann Pietrangelo

CHAPTER 28
Roll the Dice, Spin the Spinner, Pick a Card

The relapses that were so predictable and symmetrical for the last several years are no more. People used to ask me, "Are you on the way down again?" or "Are you on the way up again?" and I'd be able to answer with confidence. Now I haven't a clue. Up, down, all around.

Relapses no longer come and go with any semblance of regularity and, more often than not, I do not fully recover. Sometimes I am left using the cane and unable to drive for as long as eight weeks, and I experience brief explosions of symptoms within remissions. It's all a great big crapshoot now, every day an adventure.

While I used to experience extreme numbness and a feeling of needles and pins, it is morphing into an intense ache and throbbing that is beginning to make it onto the pain scale. Sometimes the soles of my feet and the palms of my hands feel as though they are on fire, and the sensitivity is beyond belief.

When the feeling persists for days on end, it is increasingly difficult to write. My hands seem to lose their familiarity with the keyboard, and the longer I try, the more painful it becomes.

I've adjusted to a lot of things since MS entered my life, but this is going to be a bitter pill to swallow. I finally found something I truly enjoy, and something that MS hadn't been able to take from me, and now ... this is simply not acceptable. I don't care how much it hurts, I'm not going give in to this. At least that's what I say today. But what if it persists? What if this is how it will be from now on? It's hard to concentrate on anything when my hands and feet keep screaming at the top of their lungs.

The one talent I always had – sleeping well – is no match for this either. C'est la vie.

It is the emergence of this state of being that allows me to comprehend the push for medical marijuana, end-of-life issues, and chronic pain. When those topics are viewed hypothetically, it is easy to pass judgment and clearly differentiate between black and white, right and wrong. When you get a taste of it in reality, there is a lot more gray. There are so many people with problems greater than my own.

Modern medicine is a wonderful thing and I certainly would not want to set the clock back, but medicine can go too far, actually prolonging suffering. As far as pharmaceuticals go, it's obvious we've gone overboard. There's a pill for everything and doctors seem to whip out that prescription pad all too quickly. And I don't understand why medical marijuana isn't legal. The potential side effects pale in comparison to those for the prescription drugs shoved down our throats on a daily basis.

I'm very fortunate. Years after diagnosis, I still have periods of remission where I am relatively free of serious symptoms. But I've had a peek into that world of chronic pain and discomfort, periods where quality of life is a serious issue. If that state should persist indefinitely and if a little marijuana could give me brief respite, I don't see why I shouldn't have that choice. It is nonsensical to me.

At this point, everything about how we handle health care is nonsensical to me. We're paying more and more for health coverage that covers very little and, even then, our fate generally depends on the whim of insurers. I've never felt so vulnerable in my life.

My first symptoms were easy to dismiss – certainly not the kind of thing that makes you rush out to see a doctor. Jim was far more concerned than I and mentioned it one weekend while visiting with his physician father. Dad, as I've come to call him since, immediately heard alarm bells going off all over the place. He did impress upon me that I needed to see a doctor right away, but didn't get into specific theories … and least not with me.

I didn't know it until after the diagnosis was confirmed, but apparently, Dad told Jim that very day that my symptoms, as inconsequential as I thought they were, were consistent with MS.

Dad was still practicing until his retirement at 81 years old. The last few years of his career were spent visiting homebound elderly patients who, if not for him, would find a doctor's visit all but impossible. He was a good old-fashioned, hands-on healer who made a difference in the lives of his patients.

Little did I know what was to come or how dramatically my life would change after that weekend. But it doesn't stop there. I don't have MS alone. Besides being a person with MS, I am a sibling, a spouse, a parent, a friend, a co-worker. I count on a lot of other people and they count on me. MS has spread its tentacles out and affected everyone in my life in largely inconsequential ways, and in profoundly significant ways – emotionally and financially.

There have been private moments when I wonder what I might have done to cause my MS. Medical science has yet to isolate the exact cause of MS, although there are more than enough theories to go around. The most prevalent of these is that there is a genetic predisposition coupled with an environmental cause. I have no control over my genetics, but I can't help but notice that both migraines and MS are absent from any of my known relatives. As for environment, I have lived separately from my siblings and other relatives since my early twenties, so my environment has been unique in my family. Still, to try to find some particular incident or exposure out of decades of life is like looking for that proverbial needle in a haystack.

If I did somehow expose myself to a harmful agent, I can only hope that my children somehow escaped it. I try not to focus on such things, but in the wee hours of the morning, when sleep evades me, the mind inevitably makes the trek.

I can live with this thing, but I don't know how I would handle it if one of my children were stricken. It is a thought I actively work on dismissing, again and again.

Life happens. You roll the dice, you spin the spinner, you pick a card. Then you deal with the results. Believe it or not, I find that to be a comforting thought.

As a child, I wanted the game of Monopoly more than anything. As Christmas approached, I took every opportunity to make my wish known. Sure enough, on Christmas morning there was a package with my name on it under the tree. It had that familiar rectangular shape of a board game and I was convinced that I would soon be maneuvering the thimble around the board.

Instead, I was the recipient of a game called Go For Broke. It was the exact opposite of Monopoly ... the Anti-Monopoly. The point of this game was to LOSE money! First one to lose all their money wins! Yay!

I thought my parents had gone mad, but I conscripted my siblings into service and we played Go For Broke. Against all common sense, we competed to lose money.

Why Mom and Dad pulled this bewildering switch on me I never knew. I'll hazard a guess that the store was out of Monopoly due to the Christmas holiday and Go For Broke looked similar in that play money was involved, so what's the difference? Whatever the reason, more than four decades have passed and I still remember the lesson learned. You don't always get what you want. And that's okay. It's making the most out of what we do get that counts.

Since then, I've received Go For Broke-like surprises countless times. When that happens, there is nothing left to do but play the game.

All I really have to deal with is today, and on this day, I am alive and a functioning member of society. Our marriage is a happy and nurturing one, and our families are doing well for the most part. Our health issues, career choices, and problems with the health care system are all side issues, really. We don't know what tomorrow will bring – we'll have to wait to see where the spinner lands tomorrow.

Ann Pietrangelo

CHAPTER 29
Handicapped People Steal Shower Chairs

Liz is dating a young man who uses a wheelchair as a result of spinal cord injury. It has profoundly affected the way she sees the world. The two of them took a road trip recently. Daniel, knowing his own needs, made sure to call ahead to ask about handicap accessibility and his specific requirements.

Even so, things didn't run very smoothly. The bathroom did not have a walk in shower or tub. More importantly, it did not have a shower chair, and the hotel did not have one to offer, presenting an unfortunate problem.

Liz was stunned and upset upon hearing the hotel manager's cold manner and head-scratching reasoning, "Handicapped people steal the shower chairs." It paints a ludicrous picture of people in wheelchairs leaving the hotel with shower chairs on their laps. He offered a $20 per day discount for their troubles and she was forced to go shopping for a suitable shower chair for the duration.

Liz is generally loathe to put up any level of fuss over such things, but because she felt it more an issue of justice and dignity than one of imposition, she followed up with a letter of complaint to the hotel chain. Her outrage, even over the phone, was apparent.

Personal experience is helping me to understand the intricacies of handicapped entrances and their purpose. Generally, they have a ramp of some sort that allows wheelchair users easier (relatively speaking) access. They aren't always the best option for someone like me who is dealing with limited mobility and using a cane. More often than not, it entails a longer walk and more effort than the general entrance itself. The same holds true of handicapped parking spaces. Some are specially marked to indicate ramps and adequate space for wheelchairs, but that doesn't necessarily mean a shorter walk. It is important to understand that the words "handicap" and "disability" refer to a wide variety of conditions and it is up to each of us to learn what works best for our individual needs.

Business owners should take note. Tens of millions of Americans have some form of disability affecting daily living and, as a group, have a lot of discretionary dollars. People with disabilities enjoy going out and socializing with friends and family. If they cannot enter an establishment without a great deal of difficulty, they will simply patronize a competitor.

A visit to our little local shopping mall recently got my own dander up a bit. My optician is located there, and I needed to pick up my new contact lenses, plus I needed to pick up a greeting card. I was moving with great effort that day, but was still able to trust my driving skills. I carefully planned my trip to the mall, including which entrance would be most efficient for my appointed rounds. I made a mental image of the mall, the two shops I needed to visit, and the best way to handle it in my current condition. Ours is a very compact mall and, with our small population, crowds are not generally a problem. Should be an easy in and out.

Ah, but we all know about the best-laid plans of mice and men and people with MS. There is a small section of the mall set aside for train rides for the preschool set. It generally runs in a circle in front of one of the anchor retailers. I never paid much attention to it, but on that day, I couldn't escape the train gone wild. Apparently, someone had the bright idea that the train should run freely throughout the mall. Waving and smiling little tykes were having a good old time. Cute. Cute. Cute. Unless, of course, you have any kind of disability that makes walking difficult. Despite all my advance planning, I failed to take this kiddie train's new excursions into account.

Aiming carefully toward my destination, I spotted the approaching train heading in my direction. Other shoppers crossed over or moved off to the side. I had little choice but to do the same, but at a much slower pace. Then I had to cross over once again to get where I was going.

More steps were added to my little trek, but I didn't give it much thought until I had to go back in the other direction. My legs were tiring and I was concentrating on my gait, vaguely aware of sounds from behind. Oh, no! Here comes the train again.

Toot, toot! Cute train. Cute toddler in the back. *Toot, toot!* I'm moving as fast as I can. My shoulder was actually brushing the side of the storefront and I was as far to the right as I could manage. *Toot, toot!* It wasn't so cute anymore, as I realized I was expected to move completely out of the way, which meant ducking into the next store entrance. I turned to the young driver and waved him on with a smile and an exaggerated flourish.

I didn't want to be the killjoy who ruins the fun for everyone, but when I thought about it, I realized how insensitive management was to those of us who have disabilities. At the very least, they should have trained their drivers to give way when the situation called for it. After all, it is unlikely that the toddlers have pressing engagements.

After ruminating on that for awhile, I contacted management. I was polite and simply explained my experience, suggesting that a little driver education would go a long way. I never did receive a response, but the train soon disappeared from the mall.

Liz has changed a lot lately, in part due to being on her own and college life in general, but a large part having to do with her personal experiences having a mother with MS and a boyfriend with spinal cord injury. Her assumptions about life have been challenged. She is seeing a side of things she might otherwise not have known, and it is seeping into her choice of studies and career. She wants to help people who are recovering from traumatic brain injuries. Good for her! She's finally found her passion and I am proud and enthusiastic about her choices. She is going to be a force for good in the world.

With a degree from the Rehabilitation Institute at Southern Illinois University Carbondale, she will find opportunities all across the country to improve the lives of people with disabilities. Graduates from this program end up in the private sector as well as at public agencies, hospitals, schools, and human service organizations.

Listening to her speak of accessibility limitations has opened my own eyes as well. While I know intimately the challenges of getting around when my own legs refuse to function, I also get to live on the other side of things. I live in parallel universes.

I once asked Liz to share her thoughts when she first heard about my own diagnosis. She found it difficult to put into words and said, "It's something you've really got to see for yourself." The events leading up to my diagnosis made me appear weak and run down to her, but she always figured it would pass. She never envisioned her energetic mother with a disability. She didn't mention any fears about her own odds of having MS.

She's learned a lot about MS since then, mostly because she questions me. We almost never have a conversation in which she doesn't inquire about how I am doing. "How are you? Are you walking okay? Can you drive?" And she listens patiently to my answers, letting me know that she cares.

After her last visit, she told me that, despite my opinion to the contrary, I look like a person with a disability. "Mom, I can see that you have a hard time and that things like work and transportation are a problem." Of course, she doesn't see me all the time. I'm still convinced that at times I am quite the picture of health.

There are times when I am in public when I get a strong sensation that is hard to explain. I notice people with canes, walkers, or crutches and I see the occasional person in a wheelchair. I step ahead to hold doors, or make a conscious move to clear the path for them, and make a special effort to smile. In large part, they appreciate it. But they don't realize that I'm like them, too. I am one of them.

Likewise, when I am struggling with an MS relapse, I think to myself, "they don't realize that I'm one of them, that I hold doors and help out, too." Both realities are mine. It is one of those relapsing/remitting MS mind games that isn't a bad thing. On the contrary, it's a good thing. It expands your mind, letting you not only see, but experience both sides of the same coin. At least it does for me. Despite the physical torment that MS can sometimes be, I am grateful for the lessons I have learned, and am still learning. And I'm grateful that I am still basically a healthy, active person.

Any relapse could be the one from which I don't recover. An awful lot of people with MS go on to a progressive form at some point. I could also get hit by a truck tomorrow.

As for Liz, she knows that being female and having a parent with MS increases her own chances. "I can't worry about that now," she says, but I wonder if she does. I wonder if, when she hangs up the phone, she worries. She's had a lot of tripping incidents lately and is feeling rather klutzy. She's been seeing a doctor about pains in her hips and legs, too, but we don't have any answers yet. They've got her doing a lot of physical therapy, but we're really not sure what to expect.

We dance around the subject, but I know that when we are each alone, we silently harbor fears about her and MS. Please, don't let it be so.

CHAPTER 30
"And every day I think you're a bit nuts."

It's not as if we dress like June and Ward with neckties and pearl necklaces or anything, but we do like to be presentable at dinnertime. Just because we're married, it doesn't necessarily follow that we should be slobs. Tonight is an acceptable exception to the unwritten rule.

Hair stuck to my head, shiny face, oversized cotton tee shirt, denim shorts, and bare feet, I call my beloved to dinner. My thighs are stuck to the chair and the back of my shirt is wet. Jim looks as though he just stepped out of a sauna. Not exactly dream date material, but we can be forgiven.

The temperature reached 99 degrees today and our air conditioner is on the fritz, so we're making do with a couple of fans blowing the hot air around. I grew up in a home without air conditioning, and neither my first apartment nor my first car had the luxury. It makes me wonder how I ever survived such prehistoric conditions and how I managed to get so addicted to modern conveniences.

I'm serving dinner in the dining room to take advantage of the cross-ventilation and escape the heat of the oven. Jim points out that the candles make it seem hotter (they do), so I blow them out.

We've been playing a nasty game with the air-conditioner repairman these past two weeks and it is getting old. First, he didn't show up when he was supposed to. Then he showed up and didn't have the right part. Then he fixed it ... but it was causing trouble again within 24 hours. It is hot and humid and we are losing our patience.

Finally, Jim decided to give it a try himself. After some investigation, he identified a bad part, made a quick trip to the hardware store, and restored our faulty air conditioner to working condition. No thanks to the rude repairman whose bill will arrive in our mailbox this week.

The same scenario played out recently with a plumber. Jim used to tell me he wasn't very handy around the house, but that wasn't quite true. It just took a few incompetent professionals to bring out the handyman in him. He's actually quite the jack-of-all trades.

There's a downward trend underway. I felt it coming on as long as a week ago, but had not mentioned it.

It's not that I want to fool Jim, because there is nothing in that for either of us. It's just that I want to delay the inevitable. Why put this on his radar screen before it is necessary? It might even help me a little bit, to hold on to my temporary state of denial and just keep pushing through.

By morning, I've got another small mountain to climb.

"It's time to get up, honey."

"Hmmmmm ... Okay." I have been awake for a few minutes already but haven't budged. My neck and shoulders hurt, I don't know where my left leg is, and the palms of my hands are throbbing. Even worse, I feel a migraine coming on. If ever there was a day to stay in bed, this is it, but I start the process of gathering my body parts into formation and sit up. I imagine this is what it feels like to be 90 years old.

I force my left leg into compliance and my feet hit the floor, my soles throbbing in almost perfect rhythm.

I leave the bathroom light off as I step into the shower, letting the warm water land on my shoulders, hoping to loosen them up. I fumble with my contact lenses and, for some reason, can't manage to get them in right until my cheeks are flooded with tears. Oh, it's going to be one of those days.

Jim insists on starting each day with breakfast, so I eat his offering and work on pretending that all is well. I am fooling no one, not even myself. "What's wrong?"

"I have a bit of a migraine. It will probably ease up soon." Did I say a bit of a migraine? Why do I say things like that? My head is about to explode! It is at least a level seven on my personal migraine scale, the final level before I completely lose it and have to hide in the dark. A bit of a migraine, indeed. That's like saying there is a bit of sand in the desert. I don't believe for a moment that it will ease up.

At the office, I quickly take my seat and put shoulder to grindstone. I don't want to talk to anyone and I don't want anyone to ask how I am. I just want to do my work and get the hell out of there. It is a busy day and everyone else seems to have their own problems, so I get my wish.

By 1:15 p.m. I'm grateful to be home. After kissing my husband, I generally change clothes, put my feet up, and watch *The Young and The Restless* – a supremely guilty pleasure that I almost hate to admit – while eating lunch, and recharging my batteries. Today I don't care about lunch or the show or even the article I'm supposed to write.

Jim gets his kiss and a pitiful explanation that the migraine is in full force, raging like a nuclear blast. I don't even bother to change my clothes before practically falling on top of the bed with an ice bag for my head. Smokey is nosing around, but I'm in no mood for companionship. "Get out of here!" I hurl a pillow in her general direction. It's hard to get rid of a cat that wants to sit on your chest and bump her nose on your chin, but I choose to suffer with her rather than get up to remove her from the room. It's that bad. And she's that fixated.

Jim is just across the hall quietly working while I lay here silently screaming inside my own head. I've all but forgotten the MS symptoms while the migraine rages on and my stomach threatens to revolt.

No matter how bad my MS has been at times, I always manage to make my peace with it, trying to figure a way around it. Migraines are different. My personality is lost in a fog and I cease to be me. The pain, unless you've experienced it for yourself, is impossible to describe. When it goes on long enough, it makes me want to die. Literally.

After a few fitful hours, I drag myself to the kitchen to make dinner, every step another throb in my temple. I said I'd make dinner every night and I aim to keep my word, but I never said what kind of dinner. At least the air conditioner is working.

Generally, I enjoy the process of preparing the evening meal. I particularly enjoy the task of slicing or chopping fresh vegetables. I adore the colors, the sounds, and the aromas. I don't use kitchen gadgets that help with the slicing and dicing; I like doing it the good old-fashioned way. I find it frees my mind to think things over or to sing with the radio. But tonight it's going to be leftovers from last night and the trusty canned vegetables I keep around for just such occasions. I know Jim will not complain.

As we seat ourselves at the kitchen table, I can't believe I'm even able to participate. How I am managing to function with both the migraine and MS symptoms is beyond me. There's got to some kind of powerful life force infusing me with strength and carrying me along.

I observe Jim chewing and wonder if he has the vaguest idea of the extent of my agony at this moment. From the look on his face, he has some idea. "Do you want me to do the dishes tonight?"

"Thanks, hon. That would help a lot. I really need to get back to bed."

There are pangs of guilt as I exit the kitchen, but I quickly dismiss them and disappear into my migraine/ MS fog and sleep through until morning.

With the first blush of awakening, I am aware that the migraine has dissipated and I breathe a sigh of relief and send a heartfelt thank you out into the universe.

Now where did I leave my left leg? I know it's down there somewhere. I am Humpty Dumpty and I wonder if I will manage to get myself together again.

I unravel myself from the sheets and wiggle into a sitting up position. It's a ludicrous picture, but it is my life. While Jim is downstairs doing his morning exercises, I will attempt to appear human by the time he returns. Time. What time is it, anyway? I reach out for my eyeglasses and gasp. It's 9:45! Oh, Jim must have decided that I am not fit for work today and let me sleep in. Bless his heart.

I take a deep breath and remind myself that no matter what MS decides to do to me today, it won't rival yesterday's migraine. I'm still me inside my head and that counts for everything.

Relieved that I don't have to think about work, I sink back down into the bed. Here I am safe and secure. Here I don't have to move much.

Just as I begin to appreciate the aroma of fresh coffee, Jim arrives, my knight in shining armor, with a cup of hot black morning brew in hand. He places it on the nightstand and bends over to kiss my forehead. "How're doing, babe?"

"I have no idea. Hmmm … That coffee smells good."

"Let me know if you need anything."

"Thanks, sweetheart." It's true what they say about the little things in life. "Every day I'm grateful to have you for my husband."

"And every day I think you're a bit nuts." The man has a hard time taking a compliment.

I savor every sip of coffee before I can no longer delay getting up, which turns out to be anything but graceful. My knees buckle as my feet touch the floor and I grab the nightstand to steady myself. With one hand using the bed for leverage, I make my way toward the bathroom, doing a little inadvertent two-step along the way.

"What was that?" It's part of the routine, Jim asking that question and me letting out a quiet laugh.

Sitting on the toilet, I wish I had grab bars to help me get back up. I manage well enough, brush my teeth, and comb my hair before heading to the kitchen for a piece of toast and my daily injection. Fat lot of good it does me.

I don't bother with slippers because my bare feet grip the floor better anyway. We don't have a large home, but the distance from the bedroom to the kitchen seems like light years. I pull out the stool and plop myself down right in front of the toaster and within reach of the refrigerator. I'll slap some butter on this toast and eat it without ever moving.

Before I can even think about showering, I lumber over to the sofa for a rest. Smokey hops up onto my abdomen and begins her purring routine. Fine. There's something in it for both of us.

I feel like I'm drifting off again. How long have I been laying here without movement? The soles of my feet are throbbing with pain and my palms are on fire. My shoulder, my neck, it all hurts to some degree or other, but I console myself with the fact that it's still not like a migraine. I wonder how long I can still make that comparison with the same results.

I put my glasses back on, disturbing Smokey. It's 12:30 already. I'd better think about taking a shower. Righting myself takes effort and tears begin to fall. I'm not crying and I'm not feeling sorry for myself. It's just another one of those crazy things that comes and goes in my life. Near paralysis, vertigo, trouble chewing, migraines, ocular migraines, tearing up ... the list keeps growing. It is amazing that I continue to function so well.

I think back on some of the things I complained about in my younger days. If only I'd known then what I know now, I might have enjoyed myself more. In life all things are relative. When I was four years old and scraped the skin right off my knee, it was a monumental crisis. At 19, I considered the removal of my wisdom teeth very painful. I wasn't able to get braces for my teeth until I was 20 years old. It was a blow to my frail vanity, even though I did it of my own free will, with forethought and determination.

But if I skinned my knee today, I wouldn't give it a thought. As to other little health issues I experienced, they were all temporary, all could be fixed or improved. You have a problem, you work out a solution.

MS ... that's a whole different ballgame. It's not temporary. For all the advancements in research, it is doubtful there will be a cure in my lifetime. It's a definite game-changer. If I had to have something, why couldn't it be something more ... I don't know ... understandable. Why do I have to have something so misunderstood and ambiguous? Not that I want a heart attack or anything. At least I am still alive and, for the most part, well.

Little did I realize that in just a few years, I would have to deal with something much more widely understood, but more dangerous.

Stepping into the shower I come face to face with my loyal goldfish and can't help but smile. The little plastic fish has been hanging around with me since two-year-old

Tommy presented it as a Christmas gift. What ever possessed him to choose this goldfish as a gift is a mystery to us both now, but it is one of my most treasured possessions. When I clean the shower, I also give the fish a little scrubbing to keep him clean. I want him around for a long time.

Some people have their family heirloom china, crystal, or collectables. I don't generally get attached to things. I've always been good at keeping memories in my heart, and I hate having too many possessions. But there are a few strange items, like my little goldfish, that I would hate to part with.

On a recent road trip to Rhode Island, my mother sent us home with a few interesting items that have no financial value whatsoever, but give me a connection to the past. I remember a scene in the movie, *The Sixth Sense*, where a woman is trying to sell an antique ring by telling a story about the previous owners. She explained that people leave something of themselves on their possessions. Maybe that's far fetched, but I like the idea.

That's why my grandmother's teapot has a prominent spot in our kitchen. My mother gave it to me because when I was a young girl, I gave it to my grandmother for her birthday. I didn't have much spending money, so I know it didn't cost much, but I did have to trek down to the store and choose it by myself. My grandmother was the sort who smiled a lot, and whenever I see her teapot, I see her smile.

The shower feels good, but my legs are straining and I'm concerned about falling. Now wouldn't that be dignified? I pull the shower chair under the spray and take a seat. Make-up and hair will not be part of the picture today, and I think I'll just stick with the robe at this point. My ballet-style slippers will take care of the rest.

Back to the sofa with the laptop in the hopes that a blog post will result. I have to keep shifting my position as different parts of my body hurt or go numb. I settle in with my feet on two pillows and my back to the sofa's arm. No matter how I position the laptop, my arms are killing me and there doesn't seem to be a way around this. But I'm not going to give up. This blog post *is* going to happen. So I type a few lines and rest, type a few lines and rest. It takes awhile, but I'm finally able to upload my post. Ha! Take that MS!

Right on schedule Jim takes the pulse, "How're you doin' out there, babe?"

"I'm fine. You're so sweet ... I'm so glad I have you."

"I'm not so special, I'm just checking on my wife." He doesn't get it and perhaps never will. I don't know if I'm a typical woman or not, but I know what makes me happy and what is important in life, especially now. It's not about jewelry or perfume or showy evenings out. It's in the little things he gives me every day. Love and respect; friendship and romance. It's in caring about my feelings even if it's inconvenient; it's in being more than a lover, but a friend. The simple courtesies he extends on a daily basis encourage me to do my best to reciprocate.

"You just don't get how great you are."

"You really are nuts."

Well, maybe I am, but I don't know if I could maintain a good attitude or deal with MS without him. I carefully place the laptop on the coffee table, sink deeper into the sofa, and close my eyes.

My arms still hurt and my feet still throb. I know it's going to be this way for a couple of weeks, but chances are that I'll begin to improve again after that. As long as I have MS, I'm grateful to have the relapsing/remitting kind.

It is during these relapses, when I'm unable to do much besides vegetate, that my mind wanders into unchartered waters. I am powerless to stop the train of thought or how quickly my mind races. It's almost as if some mad remote control operator is loose in my brain.

Liz is still experiencing strange symptoms. She's been to a few doctors, but there are no answers yet. One of them mentioned MS even though she hadn't told him about me. I don't think I can take it if she has MS. I really don't. That would be too bitter a pill to swallow.

I hate the state of health care and how little compassion there is for the ill. Jim and I are still hanging in there with insurance, but fear it is only a matter of time.

Tommy. I think about him a lot. He is making clear his intention to become a professional wrestler. I don't understand wrestling and never even wanted him to watch it, but what're you going to do? I'm middle-aged and suddenly decided to be a writer, so I do understand about dreams. We're both dreamers, but we're also doers. Go for it, Tommy. When your dream revolves around something so physical, time is of the essence. There's nothing worse than sitting around when you are 40 years old, wishing you'd given your dream a shot, but knowing it is too late. I will always cheer you on, kiddo. You are an inspiration.

David, that goofy kid who bit the dentist, is teaching and working on his masters. How he survives his gruesome schedule is beyond me. Shoulder to the grindstone, that one.

I wonder what's on the tube tonight. We'll probably make popcorn, but I know my arms will object to the back and forth action involved. I do love popcorn, so I'm sure I'll manage.

I hope that's Smokey playing with my head, or I'm in big trouble. She puts one paw on my left shoulder and works her way back down to my abdomen. She enjoys the soothing rhythm of my breathing and I must admit that I find her presence comforting.

I wish I could turn off my thoughts and just be for a moment. Just listen to the sound of our water fountain and the birds chirping outside the living room window. It's what I want to do, but my thoughts won't stop. *I hope Liz doesn't have MS ... a wrestler ... popcorn ... Smokey ... why is the theme song from Jeopardy playing in my head ...*

Ann Pietrangelo

CHAPTER 31
Old People in Cardigans

At least it gives you fair warning. "The moving walkway is now ending." I spent most of my life avoiding moving walkways. Why on earth would you want to stand, or even walk, on a moving walkway? I preferred to walk at my own pace, even if carrying bags and trudging through an airport. Now I not only use the moving walkway, I'm one of those people who just stands there holding on to the railing. Pass to my left, please. And try not to sigh and groan as you do.

It makes me laugh to think how annoyed I used to get with slow walkers. "Get out of my way!" I wouldn't say it out loud, of course, but I was thinking it. "Move along!" I appeared to be polite, but I was steaming with impatience inside. Perhaps it is karma that I am now one of those slow walkers in public, with or without the cane. When I become aware of the seething impatience of someone around me, I usually step aside to let them pass, and I do so with a smile.

There's something to be said for slowing down. I've grown some patience at last. When I was little, my mild-mannered grandmother was prone to smile at me and say just one word, "patience." That usually resulted in an impatient sigh from me. From this vantage point, I wonder if that wisdom of hers was also borne of personal experience.

No, life does not give you a warning, no prep time. "Life as you know it is now ending." Ah, but that's the agony and the ecstasy of life. Good or bad, you never know when it's coming. I didn't see the MS coming. I don't suppose any kind of warning would have made a difference anyway. I don't know what lies ahead, but what good would it do to know?

I'm not only a slow walker, but a frequent bench-sitter. I need to sit every now and then. Nothing tests my ability to stand more than a long line, especially one that is not moving. The forward momentum of walking, even baby steps, is preferable and less painful than standing still. So we're taking it slower these days.

I haven't done a jigsaw puzzle since my kids were little and I can't imagine what possessed us to purchase one now. We stumbled across them while shopping and somehow ended up in the game section. I guess we're going to have to plead temporary insanity. After much discussion, we settled on a 2,000-piece puzzle of the nighttime skyline of Las Vegas, of all things. When I think of jigsaw puzzles, I think about little kids or old retired people in cardigans whose kids have moved away and have only cats for company. Uh-oh. That hits a bit too close to home.

Life hasn't always been so smooth and settled. We've each weathered more than our allotment of turmoil, drama, and downright upheaval. But that was then and this is now and for some ridiculous reason we are excited about this puzzle.

The only place we can find to set it up is on the dining room table, something I am loathe to do. It upsets my sense of space and balance, but it is the only place it will fit. I hope it doesn't take us too long to complete because I know it's going to bug me.

It takes forever to locate the edge pieces and when we finally get them assembled, it is clear that the puzzle itself will take up most of the table. We'll be able to spread some pieces out on the table, but we'll have to work from the box, too. The dazzling array of lights and colors of the Las Vegas nightlife blend together, making this quite the visual and spatial challenge. This is a true test of the art of patience and I am passing with flying colors. Jim shows less endurance, but takes some small pleasure in our little adventure.

While we strain our necks, backs, and eyes on this monstrosity, we have ample room for conversation, not that that's ever been a problem for us.

I decide to tweak him. "Someone complimented my pretty green eyes today." I didn't make that up. She actually said, "You have the prettiest green eyes!"

"You don't have green eyes."

"Everyone says I have green eyes!"

"Everyone is wrong, but if you want to go on deluding yourself, go ahead."

It's a game we play every so often. I never thought I would find myself in this kind of relationship. We're definitely not The Bickersons. We just don't have it in us. We generally get along like peas in a pod. Or as Forrest Gump said of he and Jenny – peas and carrots. So much so that we notice it and comment upon it often. But we do manage to disagree often on color. I used to assume Jim had the color problem because he has a tendency to label things as "white" when they are really off-white, cream, or light beige, but it turns out that's just a guy thing. Men don't know or care about the many shades of off-white.

I've known since I was a kid that I have green eyes and Jim saying I don't messes with my self-image. I want green eyes. I will always say I have green eyes, even though my last eye appointment revealed that I have a slight color perception problem in one eye. If things really are in the eye of the beholder, I behold green eyes.

If someone were to peek through our window tonight, they would die of boredom at our seemingly mundane existence. Action-packed it is not, but it is oh, so good.

As we work, we can't help but lapse into our usual topic of conversation of late – our future. The tanking economy, coupled with our health care expenses is cause for grave concern. We've got some retirement money and investments that are worth but a fraction what they were a year ago. Our freelance status is extremely unsettling and business is rocky. On top of that, we want to move closer to family, but selling a home right now is a daunting task. Even our braided money tree died.

Our dreams and our reality are fighting it out. Our dream is to enjoy life now, while we are still young enough and healthy enough. The fact is that anything could happen with the MS. I'm in very bad shape sometimes, and with each relapse comes the renewed fear that I will not get better.

Unfortunately, the economic downturn has something to say about all this. Do we hang tight and ride the wave, hoping things will improve ... or do we throw all caution to the wind, uproot ourselves, and set off on possible adventure? In our little dream world, that adventure is possible. That's why we go online and take virtual home tours all over the world, why we attempted and failed to learn Italian (because you never know when you might buy an Italian villa), and why we are now giving French a try (just in case we end up on the French Riviera). That is why I fancy myself a writer and why Jim continues to weigh dreams against cold, hard reality. That is why we never run out of conversation. All things are possible to dreamers like us.

"That piece doesn't go there, hon." The dining room lighting leaves much to be desired and the low-hanging light fixture creates a glare on the puzzle pieces. It's a real strain on the eye. Jim's had enough and heads to the sofa, to see what's on television tonight. While he lines up some entertainment, I continue to work on the puzzle. The dining room and living room are not separated by walls, so we can continue chatting.

Over the next several days, we sporadically work the puzzle that we now recognize as a self-inflicted torture device, but that I, in particular, can not and will not abandon. I'm on a mission.

On an impulse, David decides to visit, along with two of his buddies, Pete and Pat, who have both relocated to Virginia for new jobs. With a single day's notice, but with no way to stash the puzzle, we are forced to feast in the kitchen and leave the giant unfinished puzzle in place.

It is wonderful to have the gang together at the kitchen table. The guys are grateful for the home cooking and we are grateful for their youthful vibrancy. We get caught up on their lives and can't resist a little trip down memory lane again. After dinner, the guys gravitate toward the dining room. They've been to Vegas and have lots of stories to tell — most of which they aren't about to share with us.

They can't help themselves. Pete starts rummaging through the loose pieces and Pat isn't far behind. David helps me clean up the kitchen, then joins them. Jim settles in on the sofa, not far away, and we continue to work. What kind of weirdness is this ... working on a jigsaw puzzle in the dining room with three young men in their 20's. The image of old people in cardigans is wiped from my consciousness as I hang with the young crowd. Oh, yeah. I am a happening gal.

Into the wee hours we continue working and chatting, determined to finish the puzzle that seems to have taken on a life form of its own. Finally, we call it quits, with only a few small sections to go. Even the young must admit defeat and hit the sack.

Jim and I will have the supreme satisfaction of finishing up the puzzle together after our help crew has left us for new adventures of a 20-something variety.

Ann Pietrangelo

CHAPTER 32
Bring Your Own Bowl

"Let's go out for ice cream," Jim says on a lazy Saturday morning. We don't indulge in sweets very often, and we both are in want of comfort food. We had the same urge last weekend and ended up at a little local ice cream spot. They don't really serve ice cream, but soft-serve frozen custard.

We both ordered a small hot fudge sundae and got more than we bargained for. They used shallow Styrofoam cups and enough soft-serve frozen custard that it stood several inches higher than the sides of the cup. It began melting immediately in the summer sun and I, being a slow eater, had a hard time actually eating the dessert before it slid off the sides, over my hands, and all over the ground. I prefer to eat slowly, so it kind of takes all the fun out of it for me, while still packing in the sugar and empty carbs.

I know this is not a health food, so if it's not going to be any fun, what's the point?

"I don't think I'll order a hot fudge sundae again. I don't want to have to force feed myself at that speed or get ice cream all over myself. I'll just get a single scoop or something."

A momentary silence as he steps into the shower. Then, "Bring your own bowl." Chuckles.

From the shower, "You know, that's not a bad idea. We can bring our own bowls. Why not? You've got to think outside the box, or the bowl, as the case may be."

"You want us to bring bowls to the ice cream stand?" I'm laughing, but it is a good idea. "Okay, then. Let's do it. We'll bring our own bowls."

I imagine the strange looks we might receive, but I'm way past worrying about things like that. Jim has never been one to let logistics get in the way. It is true of the ice cream treat and it is true of multiple sclerosis and our lives in general. If we let logistics get in the way, we'd never do anything at all.

"Get me a new bar of soap, would you?" I open a new bar and hand it to him over the shower curtain.

When we first moved into this house, I was horrified by the small size of this bathroom. Equally horrifying was the location of the mirror. Rather than positioning it directly above the sink, the previous owners hung the medicine cabinet/mirror about a foot off to the left of the sink. We discovered that they did this because they placed it between the studs in the wall, but it wasn't something we wanted to face first thing every morning. Imagine brushing your teeth and having to lean left to look in the mirror.

Handyman Jim quickly fixed that problem with a larger, mirrored medicine cabinet that did not need to be recessed. That problem was solved, but the pretty pedestal sink left little room for additional storage. With barely enough room for a person to turn around, Jim managed to hang a small three-shelf cabinet next to the shower.

Our morning routine quickly morphed into a thing of beauty, just short of ice dancing in its complex choreography. I shower first, while Jim does his morning exercises. He showers while I apply makeup and blow dry my hair. Then I dress while he shaves, coming back to finish my hair with a curling iron. As long as I am in remission, the dance continues without a hitch.

I used to have a much bigger need for personal space. I don't know what it is with Jim and me, but we can be together every day and never think about the need for personal space. I figure if a married couple can manage sharing a bathroom this small without killing each other, they're a good match. As for us, we even squeeze the toothpaste in the exact same spot. Marital bliss.

It is a bit eerie sometimes, as well as comforting, when Jim voices exactly what I am saying. "I was just going to say that!" is a phrase often heard in our home.

"You know, sweetheart, I love the whole idea of bringing our own bowls."

It's no different than a hundred other little things we've done over the past few years. Something isn't working for us so instead of giving up, we come up with an alternative. If it is true of the big things, it is also true of the trivial. Sometimes, you've just got to bring your own bowl.

So we order our sundaes as planned and plop them into our bowls from home. Here we sit, enjoying our ice cream in our nice white bowls from home, and I notice a couple standing around, ice cream cones in hand, chatting and pointing. At us. At least I think he is pointing at us. He is talking animatedly and appears to be looking right at us. I knew the bowls would garner some attention. That's stupid. He's more likely pointing at something behind us.

As they finish up their cones, the woman heads to their car, but the man heads over to Jim's window. Is he really going to say something about our bowls?

"I'm sorry I was pointing, but I was telling my wife about the Subaru I used to have." Oh. He wasn't pointing at us and didn't care about our bowls. It was the Subaru Outback he coveted.

"It was a great car. I put 140,000 miles on it in four years. I just loved it."

Jim smiles. "This one is ten years old. It has 120,000 miles on it and works like a charm. I hate to think of parting with it." He absentmindedly caresses the steering wheel with his left hand as he speaks. The steering wheel of the Subaru is well worn, especially on the left side. He once tried to pretty it up with black shoe polish but, as you might suspect, that didn't work out too well.

There's nothing quite like the love a man has for his car. As they lapse into that man-and-his-car zone, I keep working on the ice cream. After the guy walks away, I tell Jim that I saw him pointing in our direction but figured he was pointing at something behind us.

"I saw it to, but I knew what he was pointing at." Of course you did. It's something only a Subaru lover could understand.

Back home, I get a call from Tommy. He's uploaded a video of a recent wrestling match. Watching my son wrestle on the computer screen is infinitely more exciting than watching it in person. This way I know that he is alive and well and won't have to hide my eyes or wait in horror to see if he survives the intricate and dangerous moves.

Now that Tommy is succeeding in finding his way, I not only enjoy it, but feel myself swell with pride after his every move. He makes a very convincing "heel," which I have learned is wrestling lingo for bad guy. I wonder if acting is his true calling.

We settle in front of the computer screen and watch him in action. The crowd cheers – no, jeers – at my son, and he is playing it to the hilt. He's good. Really, truly good. He climbs the ropes and manages a back flip that causes me to hold my breath before he gets up and takes another run at his opponent.

When he first started talking about his aspirations, I don't think many people gave it more than a passing smile and a pat on the head for the kid with the dream of being a successful professional wrestler.

He's still in training and far from making the big time, but he is, without a doubt, a success. Anything can happen. He could suffer devastating injury or simply have a change of heart. Right now, though, he can see the end game in his mind's eye, and that's the all-important first step to reaching a goal. Someday he might end up the subject of a book himself, but he probably will not want his mother to write it. In the meantime, I am reading up on the business of wrestling so I can gain some insight into this form of entertainment that has eluded me thus far.

I've learned so much from my own kids. I always thought I was supposed to inspire them, but it has turned out quite the opposite. I find inspiration in them. If David can decide to trudge ahead and get his masters while teaching and supporting himself; if Liz can make peace with her own physical troubles and dedicate her life to helping others; if Tommy can face down a 250 pound opponent and look good doing it, who am I to say I can't accomplish something?

I don't hesitate to call myself a writer anymore. I know I am because I write in the shower. One of my favorite television shows of all time is *The Dick Van Dyke Show*. There is a particular episode where Rob speaks of fulfilling his dream of writing a novel. Until his wife, Laura, intervened, the novel remained unfinished due to the many interruptions of daily life and a hectic schedule. He had more than enough excuses. When Laura arranged for Rob to spend some time in an isolated cabin to write, it became clear that the only thing preventing him from reaching his goal was himself. What writer can't relate to that?

I love it when Rob justifies his lack of writing, "Standing is working; sitting is working; pacing is writing; brushing your teeth; the hardest writing is the showering!" Thank you, Rob Petrie, for validating my shower-writing.

I can't shower without ideas popping in and out. Jim tells me I've got to keep a paper and pen near the shower because I frequently run out, dripping wet, anxious to get to the keyboard to jot down my thoughts. I keep a notepad in my purse, and one by the bed. At the office, I am constantly jotting things down on sticky notes and shoving them into my purse for later use. The trouble with all those notes is that my handwriting is horrible and I often can't make heads or tails out of my scribblings. Oh, I am definitely a writer. I am just as much a writer as Tommy is a wrestler.

Sometimes you've got to forge ahead despite the odds; sometimes you've got to deal with adversity; sometimes you have to dare to dream. Rather than let life's bad moments tear you down, you've got to let them make you a better person. Sometimes you've just got to bring your own bowl.

CHAPTER 33
Happy Birthday to Us

Jim's birthday and mine are only a week apart, so we often have some kind of a joint celebration or joint gift. This year Jim has been rather insistent that we do something very special. Not only have we been through a lot these past several years, but this is a big one for me, as I mark my 50th birthday. I recall being stressed when I turned 40, but as 50 approaches I feel no such anxiety. In fact, 50 sounds surprisingly good.

At 50, I can say that I've been on the planet long enough to have earned my stripes. I have arrived. You think I don't know what I'm talking about? Well, I've been around for half a century!

We play around with destinations and dates, wondering if MS will be a factor. But our birthdays fall when they fall and we are just going to play the hand that MS deals us. Whatever shape I'm in, we are going on vacation.

There's a sweetheart deal for a trip to Key West and this time of year seems just about right. We're leaving on September 27 and coming back home on October 3. Hopefully, the weather will spare us excessive heat and humidity. It will be just the two of us and both our birthdays will be spent on the island. Our only plan is to rest, relax, and indulge in a mojito or two. Every time we see a television or movie character sipping a mojito, they seem to be having the time of their lives. All I know is that a mojito is a concoction of rum and mint leaves and I don't know what else, but it is high time I try one.

The second they open the plane's exit door, the heat hits like a sucker punch. Much hotter than we anticipated, and despite having lived in New Orleans for six years, Jim does not handle heat and humidity well at all. Knowing that would be an issue, I loaded up on a dozen white cotton handkerchiefs so he could keep one in his pocket at all times. He thought it was a silly idea, but even as we stand at the baggage carousel, he's making use of one to mop his brow. Step aside, Satchmo, Diamond Jim has arrived.

When we make it to the hotel on the famous – or infamous – Duval Street, we learn that our room has been upgraded for reasons unknown. What a great way to start a vacation! The room is in another section of the hotel and we must walk, baggage and all, in the sweltering heat. When we finally reach our room, drenched with sweat, I am ready to relax. The room is nice. It is a respectable size and has a narrow balcony. Unfortunately, the view leaves much to be desired. We did not travel to the Keys to look out over a stark parking lot. A natural view of water or assorted greenery is more to our liking, so we trek back to the front desk and state our case for our original room.

Ten pounds of perspiration later, we are finally in our new digs. This room is much smaller, but that is of no concern to us. The tiny balcony looks out over a lush green garden and a walking path. There is a large bunch of bananas hanging off to the left and for reasons I cannot explain, this makes me happy. I can't stand insects and my skin does not tolerate the sun well, but I gravitate toward nature. A splendid view of earth's beauty puts everything in a different light and makes me feel like a very small part of something so much greater than myself. Nature is splendid. The amazing thing about all this is my strength and stamina.

It is mid-afternoon and we're still acclimating to the heat, so we unpack, settle in, and put on our swimsuits. The pool has plenty of shade on one side, so we grab a couple of plush towels and choose some lounge chairs under the trees. Most of the hotel guests are worshipping the sun, something we try to avoid. The sun is particularly hard on my very white skin, even with sun block. Besides that, heat tends to exacerbate symptoms of MS. Although I'm not having any symptoms at the moment, I am in no mood to tempt the fates. I've experienced heat-induced pseudo-exacerbation before; it was incapacitating and frightening. I feel good and I want to continue to feel good, so I will content myself to rest in the cool comfort of the shade with an occasional dip in the pool and catching a few rays here and there for my daily allotment of vitamin D.

A young man stops to ask if we'd like something from the bar. The time has arrived for our first mojitos. The cool, mint-laced refreshment seems to reinforce the idea that we are on a real vacation. There are no business meetings, no social obligations ... nothing but R & R.

When dinnertime rolls around, we change clothes and decide to wander in search of food. We stumble across a Cuban restaurant and decide to give it a try. The food is delicious and the atmosphere of the restaurant is lively. I don't feel at all like someone about to turn 50 years old, and I definitely don't feel like a person who has MS. After dinner, we stroll some more and take in the atmosphere.

Over the next several days, we explore the island on foot. I am walking with unbelievable agility. The last several years have been so rough that I didn't think I would ever be this well again!

We take the obligatory photos at the southernmost point in the continental U.S. Of course, then you must see the southernmost house, the southernmost business, the southernmost apartment ... there is definitely a theme running through this island. And roosters. Plenty of roosters. Really, how many places can you go and see roosters roaming the streets and crowing at all times of day?

For us, one of the highlights of any trip is getting the feel of a place and observing its characters. People watching. The older I get the more fascinating this hobby becomes.

One of my favorite sayings is "appearances can be deceiving," and I take it to heart. Some people seem to wear their life story right on their sleeve, but I know there is much more beneath the surface. Some only hint at what lies within and some people are impossible to read.

Key West has more than its share of characters and we can't help but wonder what brought them here, and what keeps them here. Cab drivers, in particular, seem to have more than enough stories to share about how they happened to come to this place for a week 20 years ago and never left. I suppose it is part of their job to tell stories to the tourists, and they do it well. Every building, every street performer, every event has a story. Whether they are factual or embellished is of no importance.

We are soaking up the atmosphere to the fullest and I, in my state of extreme strength, am relishing each moment.

As soon as we discovered Harpoon Harry's for breakfast, we knew we would make the trek on foot every mid-morning. It's hard to pinpoint exactly what it is that makes it so good. We feel at home among strangers. There is a nice mix of locals and vacationers enjoying the simple but hearty fare. The meal is substantial enough that it will suffice for breakfast and lunch.

It is definitely a laid back vacation. Neither Jim nor I is the life-of-the-party type, preferring quiet activities to guided tours and crowds. We are so captivated with the area that we visit a realtor and add this place to our dream list of places to move. Unfortunately, the price range and cost of living are prohibitive. Then again, we can still dream the dream and take virtual home tours. We live a whole other life in our heads.

Naturally, we visit Hemingway's home and greet the descendants of his many-toed cats. Smokey would like this. It was stiflingly hot in the house and on the grounds. Jim is fairly melting and I'm craving an afternoon mojito by the pool, our new daily ritual.

The sunset celebration each night in Mallory Square is exquisite. The street performers and festivities are nice, but the actual sunset in all its splendor is a divine work of art. How come we rarely take note of this daily phenomenon? What a colossal waste.

On my 50th birthday, we ditch the pool and decide to wile away the afternoon at The Green Parrot bar. It has been around for over one hundred years and is considered a must-see for visitors to the island. For my birthday drink, I choose some kind of rum punch they're pushing and nurse it for an hour. If I could bottle this time, I would. I feel strong and healthy. No sign of MS, no sign of migraine. This place is definitely working for me. Sitting here, sharing a cool drink with my sweetheart and soaking in the sights, I celebrate my 50th year and welcome the years to come, whatever they may bring. We toast to our respective birthdays and to our many good fortunes.

In some respects, I am the typical midlife woman, a 50-year-old cliché, ruminating about where I've been and why, wondering where I am going and why. I don't really buy into the whole 40 is the new 30 or 50 is the new 40 mantra, and 50 is middle-age only if I manage to live to 100. Such philosophical meanderings don't stick with me long today. This day was meant for better things.

Eventually we stroll in search of dinner and end up dining outside under the trees and enjoying a cool breeze. Our waiter this evening is very personable, chatting us up while providing stellar service.

After we complete our meal, he inquires about dessert. We don't indulge in dessert very often, so I'm not too eager. "It is your birthday," Jim says with a smile.

While handing us the dessert menus, the waiter says, "Well, if you don't see anything you want here, I've got some other ideas ..."

"What do you suppose he meant by that?"

"Hmmm ... this all looks very good, but he's piqued my curiosity."

When he returns, Jim says, "You said you had some other ideas. What do you have in mind?"

The waiter reaches into his pocket and pulls out a business card. Looking every bit the secret agent, he lowers his voice and leans over the table as he speaks in low tones. "It's better than sex."

"Huh?"

"It's about six blocks from here. You can easily walk it. It's all desserts and it's better than sex."

He slides the card over to Jim as if it contains secret government files about nuclear weapons.

Jim looks at the card. In an equally low voice, "Oh, it's *called* Better Than Sex."

"Yes, tell them Roberto sent you. You won't be sorry." And with all the intrigue he can muster, agent 007 leaves the bill on the table and nonchalantly strolls back toward the kitchen.

Jim smiles and I can no longer stifle the giggle. Characters. This island is loaded with characters. How could we not love Key West? I wonder if there is some kind of "colorful character" test one must pass before staking up residence here. If there is, we probably have the chops to fit right in.

Jim lays out cash for the meal and, card in hand, we head off in the direction indicated by Roberto. After walking several blocks we head off the main street, as directed, onto a dark, narrow road. We don't see any other pedestrians and it feels a bit eerie. Uh. Oh. What if we've been set up? What kind of a waiter sends diners to another restaurant for dessert, anyway?

There's a small sidewalk sign up ahead. "What does that sign say?"

As we get closer we can see that it reads, "Better than Sex." So it really does exist. I hope it's for real. We pull the door open and enter a room only slightly better lit than the dark night. The room is decorated in plush red furniture and draperies, with plenty of candles.

We are greeted by a waitress who asks who sent us. I can't help but wonder if this is some kind of new age bordello and we're about to utter the secret password. She hands us a menu and pulls out a tiny flashlight so we can read it. There's a man with a guitar in the corner who begins playing. We are promised amazing desserts that will be better than sex. I order the "Kinky Key Lime Pie" and Jim takes the "Jungle Fever."

They are so large, so sweet, and so good that it's actually sickening. We can't even come close to finishing them and when the check arrives, we agree that this was quite the extravagance, but we will forgive ourselves for the birthday treat. It was delightful, but better than sex? Maybe for some folks, but we beg to differ. We'll take the real thing, thank you. It's more fun, better for you, and doesn't pack on the pounds.

We linger for a few moments, but the place is small and we are conscious of the fact that they probably want us to vacate our small table in favor of new customers. Feeling much heavier than when we arrived, we stumble our way through the dark and back into the warm night air of Key West. The long walk back to our hotel will do us much good.

Our stay in Key West, much like our honeymoon in the Bahamas, is like stepping into another world, and it's not only about the tropical weather and the relaxed atmosphere. For both of these trips, my MS has been in complete remission, and I do mean complete, as in non-existent. There isn't a soul who has laid eyes on me in Key West who would think I am anything less than perfectly healthy. Despite the heat and humidity, I am highly charged, able to walk as long and as energetically as I like. No balance problems, no vertigo, no psychedelic sideshows in my field of vision. No lightheadedness, no tripping, no biting my own cheeks or tongue. And best of all, no fatigue.

MS doesn't make much sense. Patients and medical professionals alike are hard-pressed to understand why it does what it does ... or doesn't do, and it's a different reality for all who have it.

Maybe my particular MS prefers a tropical climate. I wonder if there's any chance I could get a doctor to prescribe a small beach cottage as a cure to my MS ...

CHAPTER 34
Syringomyelia. I Hate the Word Already

The musical ringtone of my cell phone tells me that one of my children is calling. Even though I was just drifting off for an afternoon nap, that little song has my attention.

By the time I make it to the kitchen and grab my phone, the ringing has stopped. I flip the phone open and see that the call was from Liz. Lately, every time she calls I find myself bracing for some unknown crisis. Her hips, legs, and feet have been a problem for awhile now. Physical therapy helps, but the big question as to why still hangs over us. *Please don't be MS. Please don't be MS. Please don't be MS.*

We do know that some of her problems are a consequence of years of martial arts. Liz is a second-degree black belt in taekwondo, something she has been working on since she was seven years old. It was a lot harder on her physically than we suspected. David is also a second-degree black belt, but it didn't cause him as many physical problems. At one point, Tommy had a go at taekwondo, but wasn't particularly interested in pursuing it beyond a blue belt. Instead, he gravitated toward football and then to wrestling.

Physical activity is good, but fear of injury is rough on a parent. David and Liz suffered their fair share of childhood sprains, bruises, and stitches, to be sure, but Tommy managed to break his arm three times. Oh, man – nothing puts a mother in the cross hairs like bringing a child to the emergency room with a broken bone for the third time.

I hit the call back button with a sense of foreboding. "Hey, mommio!" She gives me her customary greeting in an upbeat tone.

"Hey, kiddo. What's up?"

"Well, I have a diagnosis."

Pause. I want to know … but I don't.

"Okay. Lay it on me." Breathing stops.

"Shringmla."

"What? I couldn't hear you." Darn cell phones.

"Singmalia"

What the heck is she saying? "What? I don't understand what you're saying. Spell it."

"It's syringo … something. I think it's s-y-r-i-n-g-o-something. You'll have to look it up." Oh, God. Here we go. I don't think I like the sound of this.

I grab a note pad and pen and write "syringo-something."

"What does it mean?" There is a band beginning to tighten around my forehead and I feel like I'm detaching from my body, signaling self-defense mechanisms at play. *No. No. No.*

She fills me in on the basics, sounding very much the college student. "It's a fluid-filled cyst called a syrinx within the spinal cord. It can cause pain, weakness, and stiffness, and can damage the spinal cord. Just like MS, some people are symptom-free and some have an array of progressive symptoms, like loss of muscle mass and paralysis. Sometimes they have to perform surgery."

A grenade just came flying through the window. I can see the pin is out and now I'm just waiting for it to blow.

"What causes it?"

"I don't know. Some people are born with it, some get it from injury." Maybe it was the taekwondo, maybe not. In any case, she faces an uncertain future and we've both got a lot to learn about this stupid syringo-something. I know I'll have to do my own research to gain clarification and process the news.

"Oh, Liz. I'm so sorry." What a stupid and useless thing to say. I slap myself on the forehead and look toward the heavens.

Why does she have to go through this? Why can't I do something more for her? *Why her?* And there it is. "Why her" is only a hop, skip, and jump away from "why me."

In the movies, this would be the perfect place to insert a flashback scene. This is basically the same conversation I had when I told my own mother about my MS. Back then, I wanted to alleviate her concern and I was proud of my refusal to ask "why me?" The only thing is, I'm on the other end of the conversation, and I'm not liking it one bit.

Liz is being upbeat and confident, telling me she feels so much better to at least have an answer after all this time of searching. I have no trouble believing that statement because I've been in those shoes. Finally! Someone has put a name to the craziness, validating what has been happening. Eventually that feeling will give way to questions ... many, many questions. And many mixed emotions.

She is trying to downplay the fear for my sake. I don't want her to hear the catch in my throat or the clues that I am crying, but she's not oblivious. She is so young, so undeserving of this burden. Oh, no. There it is again, the word "deserve" creeping into my thoughts. Stop it! Deserving it or not deserving it has nothing to do with anything. This is a train of thought I must derail. It is a train to nowhere.

I want to throw my body on top of the grenade to shield her, but it is not to be. She's not five years old with a scraped knee. She's a young adult with a life-altering diagnosis, and a kiss from Mom is not going to cure it.

My whole theory about rolling the dice and playing the hand you are dealt ... all my philosophizing about "why not me" is suddenly difficult to wrap my head around because if I believe it to be true of myself, then certainly it would have to be true of my daughter. The randomness of life is a fact but, as a mother, I want my children spared. Perhaps that is the ultimate selfishness.

My head is spinning with thoughts of Liz needing surgery on her spine, and the many implications of that. I am chomping at the bit to learn more about this syringo-whatever. I hate the word already. It's difficult to pronounce, difficult to spell, and difficult to fathom. It is another intruder into my personal space and I do not welcome it.

You hurt for your kids in a way you can never hurt for yourself. You have to have kids to understand that. Satellite mothering only magnifies that hurt.

When Liz was born, I imagined her nickname would be Beth. I adored the character of sweet Beth in *Little Women* for her generous and loving nature. It was a book I read at least a dozen times as a child, and read aloud to Liz when she was eleven years old.

My little girl never did warm up to the name Beth. Liz was the moniker she chose for herself and almost everyone she knows uses it. Like Louisa May Alcott's Beth, she tends toward shyness, has a loving spirit, and wants to help people. But she's also strong, independent, athletic, and very much interested in what is going on in the world. She's got a whole lot of feisty Jo in her, too.

When she was a baby, I used to sing to her, to the tune of "O, Christmas Tree, O, Christmas Tree," *"Elizabeth, Elizabeth, Oh, how I love my Elizabeth."*

After we end our phone conversation, the tune plays softly in my head and I begin to hum. *"Elizabeth, Elizabeth ..."*

My first research tells me that syringomyelia is a rare condition, even less prevalent than MS. I thought MS was confusing, but this is ridiculous. Chip off the old block, that girl. She couldn't come up with something that makes sense, something we could get a handle on, something I could do something about ...

Why her, indeed. Why her, why me, why anyone? You see it on the television news all the time, in the quaint little neighborhood where the horrific crime has just been committed.

"I never thought it could happen in our neighborhood," they always say. "I thought we were safe."

That always makes me cringe. Who do you think you are that you are so protected from the normal dangers of life? No, I still believe in my "why not me" philosophy. My daughter was dealt a card we didn't choose, but it is hers – it is ours – to play out.

Whether she deserves it or not and whether I like it or not are irrelevant to the discussion.

A second opinion would eventually confirm the diagnosis and we would have to make peace with it in order to deal with it. Syringomyelia. I'll never warm up to that word.

My daughter and I have another common bond. We're both fighting shadows. Being so much younger at diagnosis, she has a longer battle ahead, one that I am certain she can win. She will win it by living well and helping others. What her future holds medically, I cannot guess, but her future is filled with promise and I will enjoy watching her spread her wings.

"Elizabeth, Elizabeth ..."

CHAPTER 35
Then Came the Snow

I grew up in New England and spent 20 winters in suburban Chicago, so I know a thing or two about winter. I know about snow and ice and wind and cold. I know about scraping windshields, shoveling driveways, and bundling up.

I moved to the northwest corner of Virginia several years ago and have found the weather superb. Nestled in the Shenandoah Valley, we enjoy four distinct seasons, none of which are extreme. It is my favorite thing about living here. Then came the snow of 2010.

A huge storm was moving up the East Coast and by all accounts, it would be one for the record books. We did our grocery shopping as usual this week, and last night we moved my car from its space in front of the house into our single car driveway in front of Jim's. The weekend is upon us, we've got plenty of food and nowhere we have to be.

It came slowly at first, starting and stopping multiple times, but by bedtime, we knew this one was going to be substantial. I'd have to pull out my winter boots for the first time in years. As long as you don't have to brave the roads, it is a thing of beauty, framing the trees and making the world seem clean and fresh.

Before heading off to bed for the night, Jim tells me to relax and he's going to take care of the first layers of snow that have piled up outside the front door, on our cars, and in the driveway.

We can't count on MS to cooperate in any sense of the word, and of course, I'm in a relapse. I'm walking and managing to do small chores around the house, but I have no strength and my stamina is waning. The snow is already quite deep and I can't help but be concerned about his back. Jim assures me that he'll be fine, but I only half believe him. His back is as unpredictable as my MS. It isn't usually heavy lifting that sets it off, but something as innocuous as reaching for a book that will activate the first twinge and set things in motion.

"Don't worry about it. I'll be careful. If it continues to snow like this, tomorrow's going to be a hell of a day."

I kissed him at the front door and returned to the kitchen, peeking at him every so often through the bay window. Smokey, too, was mesmerized by the piles of white stuff. I'm not so bad off. I'll save my strength so I can help him tomorrow. For now, I think I'll put on some hot water for tea and enjoy the view.

I rarely awake before Jim and almost never actually get out of bed before he does. It's still early, but it is beginning to get light out and I really need to use the bathroom. Retrieving my glasses from the nightstand, I swing my legs over the side of the bed. My feet hit the floor and the throbbing begins, but I can walk better with throbbing than I can with numbness. Using the edge of the bed to steady my wobbly morning legs, I make my way to the bathroom.

We used to have a king size bed, but when we moved into this house with a smaller bedroom, we got rid of it in favor of the queen. It's not that a king wouldn't fit into this bedroom, but we both have a keen sense of space, and don't like furniture to overcrowd the room. It turns out that we prefer it, anyway. Some couples want and need space between them at night, but Jim and I prefer to stay close. We've even had occasion to share a twin bed with little trouble. When a marriage is good, it's really, really good.

I close the door of the bathroom so the light won't shine in Jim's face. I use the toilet, wash my hands, and open the window blind. "Oh, my Lord! Wow! Unbelievable!" I haven't seen this much whiteness since Rhode Island's blizzard of 1978! That storm crippled our little city for a week.

"I hear a lot of exclamations coming from the bathroom ..."

"Oh, wait 'til you see this. It must have snowed all night."

"That much, huh?" Jim sounds as though he might want to pull the covers over his head and hibernate for awhile, but he's not one to lounge around in bed once he's awake.

"You've got to see it for yourself."

I make my way over to him for morning hugs and accompany him to the bedroom window. We are awestruck by the quiet beauty of our backyard. The fence between our yard and our neighbor's is no longer visible; neither are the small shrubs or the birdbath. The larger trees and shrubs are heavy with snow, branches bending and straining under the weight. And still it falls.

In the kitchen, with our view of the street, we see mounds of snow that we can only assume have cars under them, but that's just a guess. Not even a large truck would be able to make its way down our street this morning. Our little out-of-the-way neighborhood is unlikely to be plowed anytime soon. We've definitely got our work cut out for us.

Jim prepares cheese omelets and we linger over coffee. There's no newspaper, but the electricity hasn't been affected so we check in on news reports and pictures from cities and towns all up and down the East Coast.

It's still falling and Jim starts to dress for the long task ahead.

"I'm going to help you, you know. I can't lift, but I can clear off the front steps and I can do the path to the driveway in layers."

"No. I don't want your help." He said it quietly, but firmly, as he kept readying himself for the snow.

"You don't want my help? But I'm not going to sit around and watch you shovel all this by yourself. It's too much. You'll hurt your back! I can do something."

"No." Looking me straight in the eye, he said, "Think about it. You are barely moving and getting worse. And you're having trouble with your shoulder again. It wouldn't take much for you to get hurt. Then what are we going to do? We can't get out of the driveway. Hell, we probably wouldn't be able to get help if we called 911. It will be better if you let me do it alone."

He's right, of course. He knew, even before I did, that my unearned guilt was talking, not common sense. He knew that in spite of the fact that I wanted to help, I would be unable to lift my feet through the densely packed snow, or to lift a shovel high enough to get the job done. He knew that beyond fear of injury, there was a good chance that my attempt to help would end with extreme frustration on my part.

It's the MS mind games again. What I want to do, and what I should do, are at odds. It's time to calculate the risk and reward ratio and, no, I will not be shoveling today. Jim is right. He can clear the driveway in small increments. There is no hurry because no one is going anywhere. Meanwhile, I can make myself useful with other chores around the house.

"All right, I'll work on cleaning the kitchen a bit." He opens the front door and steps out into the world of white. I find myself drawn to the window every few minutes to check on him. At times I can't see him at all, then I glimpse the tip of the shovel and a pile of snow flying off to the side. It's almost comical.

From the bay window, I glance to the left and observe our elderly neighbor at work. He can do it. To the right, children are tackling the mountains of white stuff with a vengeance. They can do it. Everyone is pitching in. Meanwhile, here I am, warm and dry, but not completely unproductive, I remind myself.

The same scenario plays itself out in summer. When we moved into this house with the great big, yard, neither of us imagined he would have to tackle most of the yard work himself. The yard has a nice lawn, lots of trees, shrubs, flowerbeds, ground cover, mulch areas, rocks ... whew! There is always something sprouting and something dying. I don't help out as much as I thought I would. Another reason we need to get a more manageable place of residence.

Once again, I am reminded of the importance of flexibility and willingness to alter plans and perceptions when confronted with a change in circumstance.

By most estimates, we ended up with about three feet of wintery whiteness. Jim broke the chore into small doses and kept at it and, thankfully, his back was in the mood to cooperate. I think he even enjoyed the excitement of it all.

Oh, you know there's going to be hot, buttered popcorn tonight!

Ann Pietrangelo

CHAPTER 36
Shades of Gray

"We have now just enshrined, as soon as I sign this bill, the core principle that everybody should have some basic security when it comes to their health care. And it is an extraordinary achievement that has happened because of all of you and all the advocates all across the country."

On March 23, 2010, President Barack Obama signed The Patient Affordable Health Care Act into law. As we watch the signing and history in the making, we want to feel victorious, but do not. We want to feel relieved, but we don't feel that either. We do, however, feel hope for the first time in a very long time.

For Jim and I, it is a victory that cannot be savored, because we did not get comprehensive health care reform. Instead, we got a patchwork quilt of reforms that lack teeth. At least we are finally taking the first steps on a long journey to right some wrongs.

Millions of people will benefit from this particular piece of legislation and, for that, we are grateful. Some will feel the effects before the end of this year, others must wait – and hold on for dear life – until 2014. Even then, lots of folks will still fall through the cracks.

As for us, even though we are still hanging on to our health insurance for the time being, this moment stings. We've always made our own way in the world; we do not abuse our health and since the cause of MS is an unknown, no one can say I brought it on myself. We know as well as anyone how seamlessly we can – and probably will – end up among the uninsured. Reform or not. Things are going to get a whole lot worse before they get better.

With this year's combined rate hike amounting to more than 30 percent once again, we are facing disaster. It is only a matter of time before we can no longer afford the premiums. As it is, we avoid seeing the doctor.

With monthly premiums now totaling several hundred dollars more than our mortgage payment, we each have a $5,000 major medical deductible, plus heavy prescription medication deductibles and co-pays. Even when the new high-risk pools come online later this year, one must be uninsured for six months before applying.

It is that six-month gap that taunts us like a monster under the bed. An accident, an illness, an unexpected complication of MS – any of these could result in bankruptcy, putting everything, even our little business and our home, at risk. After a lifetime of living responsibly and within our means, a single medical problem could cause everything to collapse.

What we wanted, and what most people wanted, was not a free ride, but a fair shake. As the bad witch said after Dorothy threw hot water on her, "Oh, what a world, what a world."

Despite warnings of the fall of civilization as we know it, as well as all out Armageddon, our basic system of insurance-run health care remains in place and even stronger than ever. The fight was really about providing access to health care for millions of Americans who have none. It won't come immediately or easily, but this is an important first step toward that goal.

When I think about the events leading up to this day, it is difficult to grasp the hatred and the anger that took center stage.

Somewhere along the way, actual access to health care became a lesser issue as other wounds bubbled to the surface.

It never should have been about President Obama and whether you like him or loathe him. It never should have been about Democrats or Republicans; right wing or left; your team or mine. It should have been about very real human beings and one of our most basic needs.

It should have been about finding a way to provide access to health care for people in one of the richest nations on earth, one which now offers this only to those fortunate enough to fall into the proper categories – like working for the right company, or working for federal or local government.

It should have been about insurers rescinding policies from people when they get sick and denying coverage to those who have had health problems in the past, or pricing people like us out of the market altogether. It should have been about states that allow these practices to continue and provide no alternatives like high-risk pools for those who are left out.

Instead of focusing on the failings of the system, we took a wrong turn and ended up talking about everything else but those failings and what we might do to improve things.

While the town hall debates were raging across the country last summer we watched, horrified, as hatred was spewed at advocates for health care reform and at the uninsured themselves. "It's your fault!" they screamed at a woman who spoke of her developmentally disabled daughter being dropped from her blind husband's insurance plan.

Without hearing the story, without knowing the circumstances, the ill and disabled were portrayed as the lazy, the leaches, the bad guys.

"Please hear the voice of the disabled," said one woman from a wheelchair. She wanted to tell her story, but the crowd was shouting her down. She wanted to tell them about her disease, her inability to pay for her medications, and fear of losing her home. She kept speaking, quietly and with dignity, while the hecklers kept heckling. She worked hard her entire life, until illness interfered, but that was lost on the haters. The woman in the wheelchair did what I'm not sure I could have done. She kept talking. She kept trying, despite the venom aimed in her direction. She was the strongest person in that room and I shall never forget her bravery.

Mean-spirited hecklers shouted at a lone man with Parkinson's disease peacefully holding a sign. He was surrounded by men leaning menacingly in toward him. "Communist!" "You have to work for everything you get!" One man threw dollar bills at him. Why did they presume he was simply too lazy to work? Or that being out-of-work should equal lack of health care?

These spectacles, played out over and over again, defied common decency. What were the bullies thinking? That these things only happen to other people? That they are somehow immune from illness, accidents, or job loss? That "those" people have somehow brought it upon themselves and deserve their fate? I guess I am one of "those" people. I have felt the indifference and the disbelief from others when the subject of health care arises, and I'm not even uninsured ... yet. It's not going to happen to them, they think; it's never going to be their problem because they are honest, hardworking folks.

Nazis, Hitler, racism, bigotry, death panels, concentration camps, illegal immigrants, and fear mongering of every sort had a place in the health care debates. How the heck did we get from there to here?

The whole thing morphed into an orgy of hate-filled rhetoric worthy of the 70's sitcom, *All in the Family*. I grew up during the era of Meathead versus Archie Bunker. Being a young teen at the time, I easily related to Michael, who was called Meathead by his father-in-law, Archie.

Michael was a champion of every cause there was. Tolerance and justice were his game, and I admired that.

Archie was a bigot and tended to spout racist, sexist, anti-everybody garbage. He never met a person he couldn't offend.

What I didn't understand as a teenager was that they were both infinitely more complicated than that.

As a mature adult, I came to understand that Archie (along with all the other Archies of the world) wasn't the one-dimensional monster I saw when I was younger. He actually had some admirable qualities, like a serious work ethic and a desire to protect and provide for his family. I even began to see that he came to his views on race, religion, gender, and sexual orientation out of pure ignorance, not that I accept that as an excuse. Rather than hate him, I came to feel sorry for him.

I also revised my view of Michael (and all the Michaels of the world.) His belief in equality was mirrored by his actions and I respect that. But he was lacking in many ways. He blatantly and repeatedly disrespected the man who provided a roof over his head and food on his plate so he could continue his education and pursue loftier goals. He didn't appreciate the hard realities and limitations of Archie's life.

If either of those fictional characters had stopped shouting and accusing long enough to listen to the other, they could have resolved many of their differences. New day, same old problem.

We became Meathead and Archie all over again. Shouting over each other and doing our best not to listen to a contrary point of view. Loudest voice wins. It really didn't matter how you got in one camp or the other. Shades of gray got lost in the black and white of it all and you were either in the reform camp or the anti-reform camp. Good versus evil, depending upon your point of view. You're either with us or you're with them – the others. Common ground was nowhere to be found.

How quickly things can change in life. Even the very ground beneath us cannot be counted on for support. In a heartbeat, "we" can just as easily become "them." It's all about shades of gray.

The television characters are forever lost in the moral issues of the 1970s, never allowed to grow wiser. We real human beings should have come further than that.

The scars will not heal any time soon, but maybe someday we can actually focus on a fairer system of health care.

CHAPTER 37
Charting the Future

"**Ann!** Ann!" Glancing around, Ann spotted the haggard-looking old woman who was gaining on her at frightening speed. Hair flying in the wind, pretty, young Ann frantically urged her horse faster and faster through the winding mountain trails. She finally reached the safety and comfort of her family, never learning the identity of her terrifying pursuer.

Decades ago, I enjoyed this haunting episode of Rod Serling's *Twilight Zone*. From the series that always ended with a twist and a lesson, this particular story made a lasting impression on me. Maybe it was because the lead character and I share a name.

Ann was 19 years old and about to make a major life decision, one that for all appearances was the right one, but that would eventually cause great heartache.

The twist was that the "old" woman she encountered while out riding was herself ... her 40-year-old self, desperately attempting to alter the course of her own history. With no future to speak of, she was doomed to spend the remainder of her days mourning the mistakes of her youth and vainly trying to turn back time.

As for the lesson, the older Ann knew she made a mistake, but hadn't learned from it, never figured out how to focus on what was ahead of her rather than what was behind her. She simply wanted a do-over, a chance to go back and change her course altogether. The younger Ann was playing "hear no evil."

Back in chapter one of this book I wrote, "We could look at this as one of those fork-in-the-road scenarios, but life's not really as simple as all that. One decision begets another, and there's always another fork to choose." I still believe that.

Forty-year-old Ann would have been better served had she taken the reins and rode off in an entirely new direction rather than treading the same old path to nowhere. Had she learned from her previous errors and determined to move forward, she could have discovered strengths and talents she never knew she possessed. Alas, she is doomed to languish in a sea of regret.

If I could give some advice to my 19-year-old self, what would it be? Would I ... could I save myself from the youthful mistakes I made? Would I have even listened? No ... I think not. Perhaps we are destined to learn the hard way, alone and in our own time. Certainly, I'm not one to dwell on the decisions I've made in the past. I've chosen to learn – to grow older and wiser rather than just older.

How about 40-year-old me? Would she be a willing listener? Definitely. At 40 years old, I knew that my journey was far from over. My mistakes served as hard-won lessons in life, lessons which I took to heart. So much yet to do and learn.

From my vantage point now, I enjoy hearing of the experiences of other women my age, as well as older, wiser women. If I should encounter my 60-year-old self, I will make it a point to stop and hear her out. Even so, I am not sure I would change my decisions. After all, my 60-year-old counterpart and her wisdom would be the result of those decisions.

Idling at a red light one morning, I observe an elderly couple slowly making their way down the street, hand in hand. Her head is tilted slightly toward his and they move in perfect synchronization. I am mesmerized.

They are to my left, heading forward, so I never see them from the front, but I imagine faces that tell of lives well-lived and contented smiles. I am drawn to them by their apparent closeness.

I wonder if they have been married for 50 years, or if they are just beginning a courtship; what their morning was like and where they are headed; what hardships they have endured and how they've kept their love alive. If there is one thing I've learned from the past, it is that the number of anniversaries we have means little. It is how we spend that time together that matters, and it matters greatly.

The couple walks out of my field of vision in a matter of moments, never knowing how deeply they touched the life of this stranger.

I like to imagine an elderly version of Jim and me, strolling hand in hand. I like to think we are walking toward a family gathering, possibly celebrating a grandchild's accomplishments or impending nuptials. I hope we live long enough and healthy enough to enjoy those things. I hope, however long we live, we never stop dreaming.

We don't know how MS will impact that vision, but MS is just one small plot line of the chapters yet unwritten. Ten years ago, neither of us could have imagined the twists our lives took to get us here. We have no idea what lies ahead. Life will surely test us again and again, in ways we cannot conceive at this moment.

This is not a storybook romance that ends with us walking off into the sunset together. This is real life — cold, hard, wild, and wonderfully unpredictable in its joys and sorrows. I can only hope that we experience them together.

We both carry a fair amount of baggage from the past. Unlike some of the stories I tell my children, some of what constitutes this baggage is far from amusing. The choices I made as a younger woman, good, bad, and everything in between, are some of the very things that have influenced who I am today, and who I hope to become.

The last few years have been a hard teacher, but many things have come into focus. Total demolition gave way to greater insights than I ever thought possible. Change takes a willingness to risk failure. So does love. Jim and I have weighed risk and reward and taken risks when the reward was deemed worthy.

Life is an accumulation of our experiences. The longer we live the more varied those experiences become and the more baggage we accumulate. We owe it to ourselves to embrace our past and our present, for they both play an integral role in how we chart our future.

It boggles the mind to think how one step in this direction or that changes everything. Every decision, wrong or right, leads us to our own future, but there are always unknown variables at work, and we've got to deal with those as we go.

It would be interesting to hear what 70-year-old me might have to say about all this. Somehow I have the feeling that she's not chasing me and trying to alter the course of our life. I like to think she's smiling and nodding in approval because she knows what's coming and I've given her many more stories to tell.

So, why a memoir? I'm not famous, nor is my story particularly unusual.

Multiple sclerosis has been the topic of many books, including those penned by celebrities, and my life is far from extraordinary.

Mine is a simple story of an ordinary life that will resonate with people who have multiple sclerosis, or those who love someone who does.

This is what happens behind closed doors when we remove our public faces and spend the night with MS. Still, it is only my story, not your story, or THE story of MS.

This is a middle-aged woman's story, a group that has never had it so good. We are freer than any generation before us to continue living life to the fullest. Lots of us have health problems by this time. How we choose to deal with them and forge ahead is something we can and should share with others.

This is, of course, not my whole story, but a carefully chosen portion that I felt was worth telling. Some events and people in my life during this time period are intentionally excluded to protect the privacy of others, or to keep from straying from the core topics.

My husband and children were gracious enough to allow me to include them, but this book is written entirely from my own personal vantage point. They are each multi-dimensional and complicated human beings in their own right, with stories of their own that are not mine to tell.

"When you have your health, you have everything." How many times have you heard that one? The young and healthy, and even the temporarily ill, can easily lose sight of that basic truth.

Whatever our religious beliefs or spiritual longings, while we are here, we are inextricably linked with our physical bodies. We must depend upon them to carry us through this life.

Once visited by a chronic illness, the truth quickly becomes clear. There is no replacement for the health we so easily take for granted. Good health and life are fleeting, but love and humor trump all. Every second matters!

A serious illness does not automatically endow us with *Tuesdays with Morrie* wisdom or *The Last Lecture* poignancy. We are, all of us, a work in progress.

My online writing and advocacy for health care and for people with multiple sclerosis opened portions of my life to people I will never meet, and I have many concerns about that. I'm not everything they think I am, but at the same time, I am more than they think I am.

I am weak and strong. I am pessimistic and optimistic, a realist prone to occasional flights of fancy. Despair and worry, elation and humor all have a place in my life.

I'm going to go out on a limb and assume the same is true of most people. If you judge yourself by the public face of another, you likely will not live up to your own expectations. Assume the other guy is as splendidly human and as flawed as you are. Learn from their success and teach them about yours. Be candid about your own foibles and laugh at yourself.

Don't ever be so grown up that the child inside you dies. Mine is alive and well, eager to see around the bend. She will know more health scares and hardships, but they will be tempered by love, growth, gratefulness for the simple joys, and humor ... always humor.

When you get right down to the every day facts of life, what makes us different from each other is less important than what makes us similar.

We are individuals, but we do not live in isolation. What we do individually has an impact on others and on the world around us. I hope my impact is a positive one.

AFTERWORD

The spring and summer of 2010 were particularly sweet. Enjoying the longest sustained remission from MS since onset, I was energetic and largely symptom free. I danced and played and openly gushed with proclamations of good health. I never felt better in my life! Just as you might expect from a soap opera script, that exuberance preceded bad news.

While blogging for Breast Cancer Awareness Month 2010, I was unaware that an aggressive and fast-growing tumor was growing inside my own right breast. A short time after completing this manuscript, I was diagnosed with triple-negative breast cancer. This was one train I didn't see coming until it hit me.

I discovered the lump on October 14 and by November 10 my body was forever altered, but my life was intact. Sometimes life is like that. That old game spinner just landed on my square again.

The best advice I can impart to others is that if you feel a lump or other change to your body, do not hesitate to sound the alarm. The speed at which we sought medical care, and the speed at which that care was given, literally saved my life. Not that the battle is over, because it's not.

With surgery behind us and an intensive long-term treatment plan in progress, we are extremely grateful to have found an empathetic and compassionate medical team. What the future holds is not for us to say, but Jim and I are up to this new challenge. Our realistic yet romantic souls are none the worse for wear. Wherever this road leads, we shall travel it together.

We were not a couple who needed a wake-up call. We have been grateful for each day that we are able to share our love and for all our good fortune. We were – and still are – a couple who feel and express our appreciation for each other liberally.

If there was one thing we may not have previously understood, it is that we are not alone. We may be geographically separated from family, but when the storm hit, all hands were on deck. We learned we have a strong support system, one that would never leave one of their own behind enemy lines. Love is everything – and we have an abundance.

I am alive. Gloriously alive! I am functioning and loved ... and yes, I still have many more stories to tell.

About The Author

Ann Pietrangelo is a freelance writer. She and her husband, Jim, are partners in WebCamp One LLC, a full-service website design, management, and development company. They continue to work and play and appreciate each and every day. Visit Ann at AnnPietrangelo.com or email her at writer@webcampone.com.